How to Lose Weight Without Effort

Part 1: Estrogen Releases FAT

Part 2, Peptides Dissolve FAT

Nick Delgado

PhD, ABAAHP, CHT

How To Lose Weight Without Effort

How To take immediate control of your physical, mental and emotional well being

Nick Delgado, PhD, ABAAHP, CHT

Published by Solutions Press
ISBN: 979-8-9930370-3-5
Printed in the United States of America

This book is not intended to provide medical advice or to take the place of medical advice and treatment from your personal physician. Readers are advised to consult their own doctors or other qualified health professionals regarding the treatment of their medical problems. Neither the publisher nor the authors take any responsibility for any possible consequences from any treatment, action or application of medicine, supplement, herb, or preparation to any person reading or following information in this book. If readers take prescription medications, again, they should consult with their physicians and not take themselves off medicines to start supplementations or a nutrition program without proper supervision of a physician.

We do not directly endorse any company or product. We align with strategic partnerships to promote wellness, prevention, and education, the triad necessary for lifestyle medicine. There may be areas of conflicting or promising data between modern medicine and holistic therapies, proof that more studies are needed. Final conclusions may be challenging given the scarcity of information, limitations in research design, and flawed data. We present our interpretation of just some of the existing data.

The dosing of peptides and peptides still in clinical trials mentioned in this book are currently under review. It is a fact that the body produces over 700,000 peptides to function properly, which decline with age.

Many social media influencers selling peptides are new to peptide research and are not reliable sources.

Individuals obtaining peptides from websites or manufacturing facilities must understand that the statement "Not For Human Use" indicates that there is insufficient information for safe use.

There is a risk even with amino acid peptides natural to the body, one must proceed with caution and be wary of the statement "My Body My Research.

The information in this book is not intended as medical advice. The decision to use peptides and specific dosing must be made under the care of a qualified doctor.

Table of Contents

Overview 7

About the Author 15

Introduction 17

Part One The Silent Epidemic of Estrogen Dominance........20

Chapter One: What is Estrogen Dominance 21

Chapter Two: Why Estrogen Dominance Is So Prevalent .23

Chapter Three: Putting Together the Puzzle— Assess Your Symptoms 26

Part Two The Sources of Excess Estrogens 32

Chapter Four: Food and Drink 33

Chapter Five: Environmental pollutants 36

Chapter Six: Health factors 38

Part Three The Delgado Protocol 45

Chapter Seven: Detox Your Environment 46

Chapter Eight: Supplements 48

Chapter Nine: Diet 52

Chapter Ten: Lifestyle changes 57

Part 4 Introduction To Peptides 64

Segment One: Introduction to Peptides 69

Segment Two: Oral Peptides (Simplified Guide and Deep Dive)..74

Segment 3: Injectable Peptides (Expanded Guide)..........84

Segment 4: Additional Peptides (Educational Purposes Only) 90

Segment 5: Expert Insights from the Delgado Video Channel..95

Segment 6: Building Your Personalized Peptide Protocol 100

Segment 7: Advanced Peptide Protocols and Case Studies 108

Segment 8: Advanced Applications and Future Directions of Peptide Therapy..114

Segment 9: The Future of Peptide Therapy and Emerging Applications..126

Segment 10: The Future of Peptide Therapy — Unlocking Human Potential 134

Marketing and Publicity..164

Book Titles that motivated me to write this book.............165

Overview

Imagine this: you wake up feeling off, drained, maybe even irritable. You brush it off, thinking it's stress, lack of sleep, or just "one of those days." But what if this feeling, this constant undercurrent of unease and exhaustion, is actually tied to an unseen issue—a hormone imbalance that's stealthily becoming one of the most pervasive health concerns of our time?

Estrogen. You might picture it as the "female hormone," involved in the menstrual cycle or something that might make women feel "hormonal." But here's the twist: estrogen, when it builds up in excess, can turn into a silent disruptor, creating what we call "estrogen dominance." And it's not just affecting women. Men, teenagers—even children—are seeing its effects, and it's happening at a staggering rate.

This isn't just about hormones acting out of balance. Estrogen dominance is a condition that affects nearly every aspect of your health, from your energy levels and mood to your weight and even your long-term disease risk. It's a ticking clock, quietly altering our bodies in ways the medical community is only beginning to understand.

What's worse? Standard blood tests often miss the mark when it comes to detecting this imbalance. That's why understanding and assessing your symptoms is crucial. The good news is, there's a proven 30-day protocol that can help restore balance, designed to address the root causes that lead to these seemingly disconnected symptoms. With this approach, you'll also uncover the hidden sources of estrogen around you—in your food, your home, even the environment—so you can create a foundation for long-term, radiant health.

Don't let this silent imbalance go unchecked. Learn why everyone—men, women, and teens—should care about their estrogen levels and take action today. Your health deserves nothing less.

In the quiet balance of life, every element holds its place. Estrogen, a hormone essential for both men and women, is no different—it has its purpose, its role in the delicate harmony within us. Yet in the modern world, this balance is tipping, as the flow of estrogen becomes unbound. Like water overflowing its vessel, estrogen in excess spills into our lives, seeping into our foods, our medicines, our products, and even our environment. The result? Many of us are unknowingly carrying the weight of this **estrogen dominance**.

Imagine, if you will, the quiet stillness of a pond. For women past thirty-five, half may already find their inner waters disturbed by this imbalance, without a single ripple of awareness. And men, too, who walk their path with strength, are quietly affected. Dr. Ron Klatz, of the American Academy of Anti-Aging Medicine, speaks of estrogen dominance as "the most prominent health issue affecting American men ages 20 to 65."

Estrogen interferes with our love life. Men age 20 to 30 have not made love to a woman in over 3 years in more than 75% of fertile men, losing complete interest. Even the young are not untouched. Teens feel the sway of this imbalance, reflected in rising rates of obesity and the inflamed skin of acne—a physical expression of inner disharmony.

Yet despite its reach, estrogen dominance is rarely seen, often overlooked. To see it, to recognize it, is to take the first step toward restoring balance. Symptoms that seem scattered—a restless mind, fatigue, cold hands, sleepless nights, or the aching cycles of PMS—may all be whispers of this imbalance. Each symptom, if we listen, is an invitation to return to center, to shed what no longer serves us.

If we do not heed these quiet calls, estrogen dominance accelerates our aging, as the very essence of our vitality fades.

We see it in wrinkles, the slowing of the body, and the diminishing spark within. More gravely, this imbalance intertwines with the roots of illness—autoimmune disorders, heart disease, and the shadow of cancer. Researchers have long known that estrogen weaves its threads through breast, prostate, ovarian, and uterine cancers. Now, they begin to see its subtle hand in other forms of killer cancers, too—a reminder that all things, when out of harmony, create discord.

In addressing this imbalance, we step toward harmony, reconnecting with a more natural state of being. When we recognize and release excess estrogen from our lives, we return to balance, and in that balance, we reclaim a life of vitality, peace, and clarity.

The rise of deadly diseases—obesity, cancer, infertility—is no coincidence. Hidden within our environment are substances called endocrine disruptors that impact estrogen levels. These toxic agents are everywhere: in pesticides, fungicides, herbicides, even in our water supply, which is tainted by industrial coatings, agricultural run-off, and household products. We encounter them daily in takeout containers, plastic cutlery, paints, adhesives, canned foods, carpets, and even in items within our homes like no-iron sheets, mattresses, and cosmetics. It's almost impossible to avoid exposure, and the cumulative effect is devastating.

What's worse, escaping it isn't as simple as hiding inside your house. Many household items are steeped in these estrogen-mimicking compounds, from flame-retardant-laden mattresses to water contaminated with excess estrogen from runoff. And when it comes to diet, the dangers intensify—meat and dairy alone often deliver up to **10,000 times more estrogen** than what's found in the water supply.

If I sound alarmed, it's because I am. Estrogen dominance is a silent epidemic, slowly infiltrating our bodies and affecting our health—but it's 100% treatable and reversible. The first step? Recognizing it. Once diagnosed, with awareness of the environmental and dietary sources of estrogen, you can take control. Recovery and long-term maintenance are achievable.

After years of research and working with some of the top names in health—like David Zava, PhD, Dr. T. Colin Campbell, Michael Greger MD, as well as I honor those no longer with us, Nathan Pritikin, Dr. John McDougall, Dr. Stephen Sinatra, and many others—I've developed a comprehensive protocol that can reverse estrogen dominance. I've helped patients regain hormonal balance, leading to profound changes in their lives: acne clears, fertility returns, weight drops, and symptoms of estrogen-linked conditions recede. Those who embrace this protocol find they can turn back the clock, often restoring blood work to youthful levels.

I've traveled globally, speaking to over 100,000 people, sharing this vital message on stages from Japan to South Africa. Through interviews with health influencers like Ben Greenfield and Dr. Drew, I've reached even more, spreading awareness of how critical it is to address this overlooked factor in health.

Yet, despite these efforts, conventional medicine often fails to connect the dots between estrogen and today's health epidemics. Testing protocols are outdated, recognizing only three types of estrogen when there are over forty. Standards for "normal" estrogen levels are based on an increasingly unhealthy population, meaning many are falsely reassured that their levels are fine.

The solution is education and action. By understanding and addressing estrogen dominance, we can make informed choices that protect our health. Let's sound the alarm and bring attention to this global issue—so that everyone, everywhere, has the opportunity to reclaim their health and well-being.

I've devoted myself to finding and collaborating with the top experts in estrogen research because the stakes couldn't be higher. Too many people suffer from conditions that go misdiagnosed or misunderstood, tangled up in outdated treatments that don't work. Uniting the newest findings, we aim to create a lifeline for those struggling with imbalances that affect everything—our skin, our bodies, even our minds.

When estrogen levels are balanced, they unlock the gates to vibrant health: clear skin, a lean physique, a thriving reproductive system, and dramatically lowered risks for breast and prostate cancers. Yet, traditional medicine has been using blunt tools—ineffective at best, harmful at worst. Acne sufferers get prescriptions for harsh creams that only inflame the skin more. Girls are given birth control prescriptions to try and manage acne. People struggling with obesity are scolded to "eat less, move more" while their real issues are ignored. Cancer patients often face only three dire choices—chemo, radiation, or surgery—without a word on how lifestyle changes could make a difference.

Our mission through the Delgado Protocol goes beyond physical health; it touches mental and emotional wellness, too. With 50 million Americans battling acne and 20% considering suicide, and the elevated depression rates among those with obesity, our approach is about healing not just bodies, but lives. Together, we're redefining what health care can be—targeted, compassionate, and rooted in real results.

Imagine this: you're making all the right choices at the hot food bar, choosing the healthiest options available, feeling good about your decisions. But, did you know that the container you're putting that food in, or the plastic fork you're using, could actually be working against your health? Or that, despite prioritizing your sleep, the chemicals in your mattress or sheets might be disrupting your hormone balance? Every day, through the products we buy and the choices we make, we're exposed to hidden hormone disruptors—things that sneakily throw our systems out of balance.

The Delgado Protocol begins here, by helping you to take control of these subtle influences. The first step is a deep cleanse: swapping out household items, personal care products, and food containers for healthier options. It's simple, but powerful. By reducing exposure to harmful chemicals, you're already laying the foundation for lasting change, creating a healthier environment for your body to thrive.

Next comes a carefully selected range of supplements. After a quick self-diagnostic quiz, we'll recommend one or two targeted supplements to help kickstart your body's natural detox process and flush out excess estrogen. It's about creating momentum—this boost in energy and relief from symptoms can be just the inspiration you need to dive into the next stage.

Then, it's time for some simple dietary changes that deliver big results. Imagine moving from a meat-based diet to a plant-focused approach that floods your body with nutrients. Instead of processed foods, you begin to crave the flavors of whole, nourishing foods. Cruciferous vegetables, like broccoli and kale, take center stage on your plate, known for their incredible power to support detox and hormone balance. And it's goodbye to foods that are sneaky sources of estrogen, like dairy, fish, poultry, pork, and red meat.

But the journey doesn't end there. This protocol is all about creating a lifestyle that supports and empowers your health from the inside out. We focus on rewiring your mindset to prioritize health, getting the restorative sleep your body needs to detox and repair, managing stress, and incorporating regular exercise. These habits help keep your body's detox pathways open and functioning smoothly. To add a finishing touch, tools like far-infrared saunas offer extra support, helping your body eliminate toxins naturally and efficiently.

The Delgado Protocol isn't a quick fix—it's an engaging journey, a chance to regain balance, energy, and well-being in a holistic way that feels achievable and inspiring. It's more than just a program; it's a way to thrive, giving your body the environment and support it needs to feel its best every day.

You may have felt out of sync with your body, carrying the weight of fatigue, unexplainable weight gain, or emotions as turbulent as stormy waters. Each time you seek help, the solutions offered feel like temporary fixes—prescriptions, strict diets, or even invasive procedures. These "fixes" leave you wondering, "Isn't there something deeper? Something more in harmony with the body's natural flow?"

Defeating the Silent Killer serves as a guide to help you find alignment between mind, body, and spirit. It isn't about relying solely on willpower or accepting discomfort as an inevitable part of life. Instead, this book shows you how to understand your body's unique rhythm, helping you access the inner wisdom within. By learning how to assess your hormone levels and recognize their influence, you gain clarity and confidence, empowering you to form a partnership with your doctor based on trust and understanding.

This journey is also about self-awareness. In this book, you'll find self-diagnostic tools, learning to listen deeply to your body's signals and interpret them with gentle curiosity. The book guides you on what lab tests to ask for, enabling you to take an active role in your own healing, rather than placing all hope in external solutions.

The ailments that once troubled you—weight fluctuations, mood swings, fatigue, and even more serious conditions like cancer or fertility issues—no longer seem insurmountable. *Defeat Silent Killer* calls both you and the medical community to look beyond surface symptoms and recognize the interconnectedness of health challenges. It's an invitation to stop tolerating suffering and to reclaim the vitality that lies within each of us.

You have the power to restore your health, to return to a state of harmony. Defeat Silent Killer" is here as a gentle, wise guide, helping you connect the dots, heal imbalances at their root, and rediscover the peace that is everyone's birthright.

About the Author

Dr. Nick Delgado, PhD, is a trailblazer in anti-aging and preventive health, renowned for his forty years of expertise in health science and hands-on experience with clients around the globe. A certified member of the American Board of Anti-Aging Health Practitioners, Dr. Delgado is one of the world's top authorities on anti-aging medicine, admired for his pioneering approach and innovative methods. His insights are regularly featured in *Anti-Aging Medical Therapeutics*, the preeminent journal in this evolving field, and he commands attention as a global speaker sought by audiences worldwide.

At his Orange County, California, practice, Dr. Delgado consults clients traveling from across the U.S. and doctors from the anti-aging field who trust him to monitor their health. He is passionately committed to educating and empowering people through his weekly web classes, podcasts, and a constantly expanding YouTube channel, *Delgado Protocol For Health*. Over the years, Dr. Delgado has delivered more than 3,000 public seminars and is a prominent lecturer at leading health expos, such as *The Breast Cancer Summit* and *The New Life Expo*. His reach extends to an international network of 26,000 doctors, educating them through worldhealth.net, the American Academy of Antiaging online platform.

Dr. Delgado's journey to wellness was sparked by a personal health crisis at just twenty-three, when a stroke led him to transform his life. In just five months, he lost fifty-five pounds, came off blood pressure medication, and embarked on a relentless mission to inspire health transformation. His success quickly led to his role as director of the Pritikin Better Health Program at the Nathan Pritikin Longevity Center.

A living example of his Delgado Protocol's impact, Dr. Delgado set a world record in strength endurance by lifting a staggering 50,640 pounds in one hour—at 52! Even into his 60s, he led Team U.S.A. to victory at the Arnold Classic World Championship.

As a certified hypnotherapist and NLP practitioner, Dr. Delgado's approach goes beyond traditional health advice, emphasizing the power of mindset in achieving peak wellness. He is the author of fifteen books, including *Acne Be Gone for Good, Blood Doesn't Lie, Stop Aging Now* and *Simply Healthy*, his bestselling plant-based cookbook, which has sold over 25,000 copies.

For more about Dr. Delgado's life-changing work, visit DelgadoProtocol.com/Hub and Foreveryoungevent.com.

Introduction

Picture yourself in a warm kitchen, stirring a pot of rich tomato sauce. The smell of simmering tomatoes fills the air, but it's not just the tomatoes that make it special. There's the sharp kick of garlic, the mellow sweetness of sautéed onions, a hint of salt, and a splash of balsamic vinegar. Each ingredient has a role, and it's only when they're in perfect balance that the sauce becomes something memorable. Too much salt, and it's overpowering; too little garlic, and it loses its magic.

This same principle of balance holds true for your body. Every day, your body orchestrates a complex mix of processes—breathing, digesting, detoxifying, thinking. These actions are driven by a network of powerful biochemicals, the most influential of which are hormones. Think of hormones as the key ingredients that make up the vibrant, ever-changing masterpiece that is you. And just like a sauce depends on its precise blend of ingredients, your wellbeing depends on the right hormonal balance. When one hormone tips too high or drops too low, it's as if the recipe's gone wrong, and you can feel the difference.

Hormones aren't just about puberty or PMS, although that's often what people associate them with. Every person, at every stage of life, is influenced by a range of hormones. Some regulate your body's response to stress—like adrenaline and cortisol; others drive metabolism, like thyroid hormones and insulin; and a particularly crucial group affects reproduction, including estrogen, testosterone, and androgen. It's this final group, especially estrogen, that will be the focus of this book because it plays such an essential role in overall health and wellbeing.

In my years as a health researcher, educator, and coach, I've had the privilege of working with over 10,000 clients and reaching more than 100,000 participants through seminars and webinars. Through all this work, I've noticed a troubling trend:

an increasing number of people are facing symptoms linked to hormonal imbalance. And it's not limited by age or gender. In my clinic in Orange County, and the doctors I've trained with in LA, and Danville, California, Michigan and Florida we see men grappling with stubborn belly fat, hair loss, and the appearance of "man boobs." Many are worried about prostate health, with PSA test results or even a prostate cancer diagnosis. Women come in seeking relief from infertility, severe PMS, and the looming fear of breast cancer. And younger clients—teens—battle relentless acne that won't seem to clear up.

Despite the wide range of symptoms and the diversity of people affected, there's one common factor linking them all: an overload of a particular hormone—estrogen. When estrogen levels become too high relative to other hormones, the body enters a state called estrogen dominance. This imbalance can trigger a cascade of health issues, from physical symptoms like weight gain and fatigue to more serious conditions over time.

The irony is that while estrogen dominance is incredibly common, it often goes undiagnosed and untreated. And that's the real tragedy, because many of these symptoms—and even some of the more serious health problems—can be reversed by clearing excess estrogen from the body. The solution isn't overly complex; in fact, it's refreshingly simple: learn to limit the estrogen you're exposed to through food, personal care products, and even drinking water, and support your body's natural ability to remove any estrogen it doesn't need.

Mastering this balance can change everything. By understanding how to control estrogen levels, you can slow the aging process, restore balance to your hormonal system, and give your body the tools it needs to resist disease and distressing symptoms. Imagine letting go of stubborn weight, reclaiming your energy, and experiencing a renewed sense of vitality in both body and mind.

This book is your guide to doing exactly that. Within these pages, you'll uncover the steps to restoring hormonal balance, revitalizing your health, and living your life with a newfound sense of energy and well-being. Let's dive in and rediscover the balanced, thriving version of you.

Part One
The Silent Epidemic of Estrogen Dominance

Chapter One:
What is Estrogen Dominance

Imagine your body as a beautifully crafted temple—each part designed with intention, every system in balance. But what happens when that equilibrium begins to shift? At first, it's subtle, like a whisper out of tune. Over time, that whisper grows louder, disrupting the harmony within. This is the story of estrogen dominance.

At its core, estrogen dominance is an imbalance—when estrogen levels become disproportionately high in relation to other hormones, especially progesterone. Though it may sound harmless, this condition can ripple through your entire system, creating far more than just hormonal disturbance. It's a silent disruptor, with the power to influence everything from your mood and metabolism to your risk of chronic disease.

Modern research has revealed a sobering truth: estrogen affects far more than reproductive health. It plays a role in the development of many cancers, as abnormal cells often thrive in its presence. But knowledge is power—and recognizing the influence of estrogen is the first step toward restoring well-being.

A Widespread Imbalance

More than half of women over 35 are experiencing some degree of estrogen dominance, often without realizing it. Yet it doesn't stop with women. Men are also affected, with symptoms that impact their vitality, strength, and aging process. Even teens are showing signs—persistent acne, stubborn weight gain, and hormonal shifts are becoming increasingly common.

Tuning In to the Body's Signals

Estrogen dominance manifests differently for everyone, but certain symptoms are consistent. Women may notice weight gain in new areas, tender breasts, irregular periods, or emotional fluctuations. Men may experience reduced libido, abdominal fat, or early signs of aging. Shared symptoms often include fatigue, brain fog, anxiety, and insomnia. Teenagers may face skin issues or sudden changes in body composition.

These signs are not random—they're signals from within, inviting you to pause and pay attention. Your body speaks in symptoms; the question is, are you listening?

When Imbalance Leads to Illness

Unchecked, estrogen dominance can contribute to serious health conditions—breast and prostate cancers, heart disease, gallbladder problems, autoimmune disorders, and even strokes. Yet within this challenge lies potential. These conditions are not just threats—they are warnings, and perhaps even catalysts for change.

Restoring the Sacred Balance

Here is the encouraging truth: estrogen dominance is not a life sentence. It can be addressed, reversed, and healed. The journey begins with awareness—acknowledging the imbalance and choosing to act. With the right tools, guidance, and commitment, balance can be restored, and vibrant health reclaimed.

In the next chapter, we'll uncover the root causes of estrogen dominance and explore how everyday choices—what you eat, how you manage stress, the products you use—can tip the scales. Once you understand these influences, you'll be empowered to make changes that lead you back to harmony and lasting health.

Chapter Two: Why Estrogen Dominance Is So Prevalent

Imagine a serene Jesus and Buddha sitting under a tree next to the continuous river of life, radiating peace and balance. Just as he found enlightenment by understanding life's true nature, we too must seek clarity on a hidden yet significant force of good versus bad within us all: estrogen. Many people are experiencing an imbalance of this powerful hormone, but not all types of estrogen are harmful—some can actually be incredibly healing. Nearly 40 types of estrogen flow through us, and like yin and yang, some support our vitality while others can disrupt it. Among the "good" estrogens, 2-hydroxyestrone stands out. It's like the gentle sage of the hormone world, guiding our body toward health by promoting apoptosis, the peaceful process of removing unwanted cells, protecting us from illness. This kind of estrogen strengthens our immune system, invigorates our mind and body, and even preserves our bones, helping us age gracefully.

Balance is the key. Not all estrogens are equal, and reducing them all isn't wise. Instead, we must protect our levels of beneficial estrogen, crucial for both men and women at every age. The problem lies with the other thirty-nine forms, some of which disrupt our body's harmony. So where does this imbalance come from, and how can we find our way back to balance?

The Weight of Our Environment

Our modern world is flooded with xenoestrogens—foreign estrogens that enter our lives subtly but impactfully. Imagine you're leaving home, only to be surrounded by invisible sources of these disruptive hormones. Car exhaust, industrial chemicals, even the film on your receipts—these are daily exposures. Xenoestrogens also reside in our homes, tucked within plastics, soaps, cleaners, furniture, and carpets, quietly contributing to estrogen dominance.

The Cycle of Body Fat and Estrogen

Fat cells store an enzyme called aromatase, which produces estradiol—a very potent form of estrogen. While we need some of this hormone, too much of it can lead to toxic effects, fueling fibroid tumors, cancer, and weight gain, creating a self-perpetuating cycle. Think of body fat as a storage of imbalance, where excess estrogen thrives and multiplies.

Food and Drink: Hidden Culprits

Each bite and sip plays a role. Pesticides on produce and the hormones in conventionally raised meat introduce xenoestrogens into our systems. Fatty foods can even convert good estrogen into its harmful counterparts. Even water and beverages can tip the scale—tap water, coffee, alcohol, they all add to the estrogen load, pushing us further from harmony.

The Influence of Birth Control

Most birth control pills work by suppressing progesterone, allowing estrogen to dominate. This effect not only impacts women who take contraceptives but also makes its way into our water systems through runoff. As if unknowingly, we drink in the remnants, further fueling imbalance.

Age and the Shift Toward Estrogen Dominance

Age naturally increases estrogen levels, especially with the silent presence of xenoestrogens. By thirty-five, many people already experience some degree of estrogen dominance.

Without intervention, this imbalance only grows as the years pass.

The Weight of Stress

While stress doesn't directly add estrogen, it throws our hormones off balance. Chronic stress drains our adrenal glands, weakening their ability to produce progesterone, the hormone that balances estrogen. Even if estrogen levels stay the same, a drop in progesterone tips the scales, leading to imbalance.

Despite the abundant causes of estrogen dominance, there's another reason why it has gone unnoticed for so long: the limitations of traditional medicine. For years, doctors only measured three of estrogen's nearly forty types. As a result, many forms of estrogen went undetected. Now, a new wave of anti-aging and lifestyle medicine experts, like myself, are using advanced methods, like urine analysis, to get a fuller picture of hormone ratios.

Finding harmony in our body's chemistry is much like the journey toward inner peace. By understanding estrogen and the hidden ways it can disrupt or support us, we can take steps toward restoring balance, health, and vitality—finding our own place of stillness amid the chaos of modern life.

Chapter Three: Putting Together the Puzzle—Assess Your Symptoms

What's Your Estrogen Dominance Quotient?

Estrogen dominance might be silently influencing your life, slipping into places you wouldn't expect—from your skin to your mood to your digestion. If you've ever felt like something's just "off," maybe it's time to uncover if hidden hormone imbalances are at play. To help connect the dots, we've crafted a self-assessment that'll give you a snapshot of your estrogen landscape.

This isn't an exhaustive diagnostic tool; instead, it's a guiding light, pointing you toward possible symptoms associated with estrogen dominance. Later on, we'll explore how you can work with a healthcare provider to determine your exact levels and make informed decisions. This journey is about finding balance, understanding the signals your body sends, and regaining control over your health.

Discovering Your Estrogen Footprint

Place a check beside each statement that rings true for you. Let's peel back the layers and see if estrogen dominance might be shaping your life in unexpected ways.

Physical Appearance

Does any of this sound familiar?

Mild acne

Severe acne

Tiny red moles on your torso

Red spots on your tongue

Flabby muscles

Excess belly fat

Excess fat on hips or buttocks

Enlarged breasts

Wrinkles

Premature or rapid aging

Thinning hair

Hair loss on top of head

Pale complexion

Cellulite on thighs and buttocks

Mental Health

Is your mind feeling like it's clouded or weighed down?

Brain fog/lack of mental clarity

Poor memory

Depression

Feeling stressed out

Feeling overly emotional

Addictions to drugs (prescription or otherwise)

Over-reliance on alcohol

Chronic headaches

Physical Function

Does your body seem to fight you when it should flow?

Poor immune system (frequent colds and illness)

Low libido

Difficulty achieving orgasm (female) or erection (male)

Low testosterone

Low energy
Insomnia
Digestive problems
Constipation
Hot flashes
Difficulty falling asleep with slight light or noise
Cravings for sweet or spicy foods
Hunger, even after eating
Fatigue that comes on strong after eating
Cold hands or feet
Dependency on caffeine to make it through the day
Dizziness after standing up
Inflexibility
Declining strength
Sun sensitivity
Slow wound healing or easy bruising
Difficulty urinating
Dry eyes
Dry mouth

Menstrual Symptoms

Ladies, do you experience:
Heavy menstrual flow
Irregular menstruation
Menstrual cramps
Premenstrual bloating/water retention
Premenstrual breast tenderness
Premenstrual headaches
Premenstrual mood swings

Health Conditions

Some conditions could signal estrogen dominance at work. Do you have:

Anxiety or panic attacks

Arthritis

Cancer

Cystic or lumpy breasts

Depression

Diabetes

Fibroids

Endometriosis

Heart disease

High blood pressure

Infertility

Insulin resistance

Polycystic ovary syndrome

Prostate problems

Thyroid problems

Tumors

Weight problems

Contraceptives and Hormone Therapy

Are you using:

Hormone replacement therapy

Oral birth control

Spermicide

Age Insight

Each decade, our bodies undergo changes in hormone levels.

Give yourself one checkmark for each full decade of life:

Teens

Twenties

Thirties

Forties

Fifties

Sixties

Seventies

Eighties

Nineties

Diet Choices

Hormones are influenced by what we eat. Consider how much of the following you consume daily:

Alcohol: ______

Canned foods: ______

Coffee: ______

Conventionally grown produce (not organic):

Dairy, meat, and eggs: ______

Food microwaved in plastic: ______

Soda: ______

Soy milk or tofu: ______

Sugary sweets: ______

Score Yourself and See Where You Stand

0-24:

Your estrogen levels are likely on the lower side. However,

watching your lifestyle choices and occasional testing can help you stay balanced as you age.

25-49:

You're likely at an average exposure to excess estrogens. It's an ideal time to get tested and make some tweaks to your diet, lifestyle, and products to maintain balance.

50-74:

Signs suggest estrogen dominance. Testing and lifestyle adjustments can help reduce exposure and rebalance your body. Embracing the Delgado Protocol could guide you toward equilibrium.

75-100:

Your estrogen levels may be seriously out of sync, likely showing up as troubling symptoms or even chronic health concerns. Testing and a proactive approach to your health are key steps in restoring harmony and achieving lasting wellness.

Part Two
The Sources of Excess Estrogens

Chapter Four: Food and Drink

The Stealthy Sources of Estrogen You're Eating

We live in a world brimming with chemicals that can tamper with our hormones, but the real danger isn't lurking out there somewhere mysterious. No, the number one source of estrogen overload is much closer to home—it's in what you eat and drink every single day. But here's the good news: by simply choosing different foods, you have the power to significantly reduce your estrogen exposure.

This chapter—and those that follow—aren't here to make you feel helpless. Instead, I'm here to show you how much control you have over your own health. As we dive in, it may feel a bit daunting to uncover all the ways estrogen sneaks into your system, but stick with me. By the end, you'll have the tools and the plan to take back control.

Animal Products: The Hidden Hormones in Your Meat and Dairy

When it comes to estrogen dominance, the single biggest contributor—by far—is animal-based foods. And while it's true that many animals raised for food are given hormones to fatten them up, the real issue isn't just the additives. Animals, like us, produce their own natural hormones, and when you eat them, you're consuming those hormones, too.

One of the most potent is estradiol—a natural hormone identical in animals and humans. In fact, estradiol from animal products is about 10,000 times more potent than most environmental estrogens. So yes, your steak, milk, and eggs are bringing a lot more than just protein to the table.

Consider this: research shows that a child's estrogen exposure from a single glass of milk is 150 times higher than from a glass of water. This holds true even for organic and grass-fed options. If you're seeing more "man boobs" and less "manly muscles" around, there's a reason for that. Estrogen dominance from meat and dairy can bring symptoms like muscle loss, belly fat, low libido, fatigue, and even depression.

Alcohol: Why "Cheers" Comes with a Catch

Even if you're only a moderate drinker, alcohol can still tip the scales toward estrogen dominance. Your liver's job is to filter out substances that your body doesn't need—including excess estrogen. Beer is one of the worst because it increases estrogen levels the most. And when you drink, your liver shifts focus to breaking down alcohol, leaving those estrogens hanging around in your system longer than they should. Numerous studies link regular alcohol intake to higher estradiol levels and increased risk of breast cancer.

Caffeine: The Surprising Link to Estrogen Overload

Caffeine doesn't just give you a jolt; it also ramps up stress hormones like cortisol and adrenaline. When this happens too often, your adrenal glands become overtaxed and can't keep up with producing other essential hormones. This hormone imbalance allows estrogen to dominate.

Chronic caffeine consumption also weakens your thyroid and disrupts blood sugar, leading to increased inflammation. This series of changes means your sex hormones are thrown off balance, with estrogen rising while testosterone and progesterone fall—again tipping the scales toward estrogen dominance.

Processed Foods: The Double Whammy

Processed foods are especially problematic for two reasons. First, they reduce levels of a key protein called Sex Hormone Binding Globulin (SHBG), which is responsible for binding to excess estrogen and testosterone in your blood. Lower SHBG means more free estrogen floating around. Second, processed foods—especially those full of sugar and refined flours—spike your blood sugar, triggering insulin release. High insulin lowers SHBG and also leads to more testosterone, which belly fat then converts into estrogen. So, that snack bar or bag of chips? It's doing more harm than you might realize.

Plus, nearly all processed foods are loaded with xenoestrogens from additives and packaging, like plastic liners or food dyes. Currently, there are over 3,000 different chemicals used as food additives. Studies have found that at least 31 of these additives have estrogenic effects, and that's not counting the pesticides sprayed on so many of our foods.

This chapter is your gateway to understanding where these hidden sources of estrogen are coming from and what you can do to reduce them. You don't have to accept estrogen dominance as a given. With awareness and a few changes, you can start shaping your diet to support a healthier, more balanced hormone profile. Get ready to take charge, because by the end of this journey, you'll be well-equipped to make decisions that strengthen your health—today and for the years to come.

Chapter Five: Environmental pollutants

Imagine your daily routine: grabbing a bottle of water on your way out, unwrapping a snack, or loading groceries into the fridge. What you don't see, however, are the chemicals silently leaching into these items—and ultimately, into your body. One of the most notorious is Bisphenol A (BPA), a synthetic estrogen used since the 1960s in plastics and can linings.

For decades, BPA was everywhere—coating baby bottles, sippy cups, water bottles, and even thermal receipt paper. But in 2008, public concern surged as research linked BPA exposure to serious health issues, including breast cancer, reproductive disorders, early puberty, and obesity. Government studies now show that 93% of Americans carry detectable levels of BPA in their bodies, marking it as one of the most widespread endocrine disruptors.

In response, companies began labeling products as, "BPA-free." But this was only a partial solution. Many BPA replacements—such as BPS and BPF—also mimic estrogen and may be just as harmful, if not more so. Studies show that nearly all plastics release synthetic estrogens, sometimes from the first use, and especially when exposed to heat—from dishwashers, microwaves, or a bottle left in a hot car. Each instance increases the risk of these chemicals seeping into our food and drinks.

But plastics aren't the only concern. Our homes are filled with other hormone-disrupting compounds. Phthalates are found in toys, vinyl flooring, and plastic wrap. Flame retardants lurk in mattresses and upholstery. Glycol ethers, common in paints and cleaning products, and perfluorinated chemicals used in non-stick cookware further contribute to our daily chemical load.

Our skin, the body's largest organ, also plays a major role in absorption. Unlike the digestive system, which filters out many toxins, the skin allows direct entry into the bloodstream. Lotions, shampoos, and cosmetics often contain parabens, phthalates, and triclosan—chemicals linked to hormonal disruption and cancer. Teen girls are especially vulnerable, using multiple personal care products daily during critical stages of reproductive development.

Outside the home, the problem continues. Hormones from farm animal waste used as fertilizer wash into waterways. Dioxins—by-products of industrial processes—linger in the environment for years, disrupting hormone signaling. Atrazine, a common herbicide, has been linked to breast tumors and prostate issues. Perchlorate, a component of rocket fuel, contaminates water and food supplies, impairing thyroid and reproductive health.

These chemicals are embedded in modern life, the byproducts of convenience and industrial progress. But awareness is a powerful first step. By understanding where these disruptors hide, we can begin to reduce exposure and protect our health. In the chapters ahead, we'll explore practical strategies to detoxify your environment, strengthen your body, and navigate today's chemical landscape with resilience.

Chapter Six:
Health factors

The last area of estrogen dominance factors focuses on personal health, specifically body fat and various hormone sources like birth control pills and hormone replacement therapy.

Body Fat and Estrogen Production

For both men and women, body fat plays a significant role in estrogen levels. Fat cells store aromatase, an enzyme responsible for converting other hormones into estrogen. Consequently, individuals with higher body fat percentages tend to produce more estrogen. For those who are obese, this dynamic can create a negative cycle. Excess estrogen encourages the body to produce more fat cells, which in turn generate more estrogen, making weight loss increasingly challenging.

The effects of high estrogen levels don't stop there. Elevated estrogen can increase the production of Sex Hormone Binding Globulin (SHBG), a protein that attaches to testosterone and prevents it from performing its functions. Estrogen also stimulates the liver to produce more carrier proteins that bind up testosterone, reducing the levels of free testosterone available to the body. Free testosterone is crucial as it is the form that readily crosses into the brain and muscles, supporting energy, mood, and physical vitality.

For men, low levels of free testosterone can contribute to weight gain, decreased libido, erectile dysfunction, low energy, and depression. For women, reduced testosterone levels are often linked to fatigue, lowered sex drive, difficulty building or retaining muscle, higher body fat percentages, and increased chances of depression.

I was given an exciting opportunity to test the idea that free testosterone, also known as bio available testosterone is more important that your total testosterone. A company owned by a successful businessman asked me to test the hormonal starting levels to see if a product called "Great Sex in a Bottle" would improve libido - the interest in sex and the experience of sex in a group of men and women.

I decided to have each person collect their saliva in a tube, then 9 days later recheck the levels of free testosterone after taking the product as they reported any differences in sexual feelings or response. To our amazement the product actually worked with both men and women reported increases in desire, interest in intimacy, and the intensity of their orgasms. We had another group take placebo (no active ingredients in the capsule). The group on placebo showed almost no change in their free testosterone levels and virtually no increase in their libido or interest engaging in sexual pleasure. the group taking the active ingredients in the trademarked product called **TestroMore**TM combined with the product **EstroblockTM** experienced remarkable sexual. Vitality!

I have continued to compare the ingredients in each product I have created and compared the results as measured by lab work and reported experience. This has allowed me to formulate the best anabolic, testosterone enhancing capsules as compared to pharmaceutical and to injectable TRT (synthetic testosterone) compared to BHRT (natural bio identical hormones) while measuring changes in estrogen including not just blood levels, also during 24 urine tests to observe how over 38 different hormone metabolites can be influenced by the best combinations.

I want to emphasize, if a pharmaceutical or nutraceutical worked as well or better with the least side effects, I would embrace the sequence and doses. the most promising area of research is in regards to peptides. Please visit the website. DelgadoLabs.com

Learn latest information in this novel category of regenerative medicine where both injectionable and oral peptides are available. Enhancing sexuality, strength, endurance, mental cognition, and quite possibly longevity!

I work with many of the top anti-aging hormone experts in the world and our protocols have been nothing short of astonishing effect for men and women to enjoy a better quality of life, reach their ideal body weight, improve their relationships, and increase the capacity to perform mentally and physically on a daily basis, there by improving the productivity of their career and health.

Birth Control Pills and Estrogen Dominance

Birth control pills are one of the most common contributors to estrogen dominance, disrupting hormonal balance in multiple ways. Firstly, they suppress progesterone production. As estrogen is naturally balanced by progesterone, this suppression worsens estrogen dominance. While supplementing with natural progesterone might help control estrogen levels, this only addresses part of the issue.

Oral contraceptives also increase SHBG levels, reducing circulating testosterone. SHBG's ability to bind to testosterone has made certain birth control pills popular for acne treatment, as SHBG binds to the testosterone variant (DHT) that triggers acne. However, in targeting acne, these pills push SHBG levels extremely high, lowering testosterone levels to potentially risky lows, while causing loss of libido, decrease in muscle density and declines in cognitive function.

Additionally, most birth control pills introduce synthetic estrogens, which are not identical to the body’s natural hormones. These synthetic versions, such as ethynyl estradiol or esterified estrogens, have been linked to various health risks associated with oral contraceptives. Some pills also contain synthetic progestin, a form of progesterone that is associated with increased risks for breast cancer and cardiovascular disease.

Even after stopping birth control pills, SHBG levels often remain elevated for years, which keeps testosterone low and further promotes estrogen dominance. Birth control pills are associated with risks of breast cancer, cervical cancer, strokes, heart attacks, migraines, and infertility, among other health concerns.

Interestingly, many people take birth control pills not just to prevent pregnancy but to manage irregular periods or acne. Unfortunately, these pills don't address the root cause of such symptoms, which is often estrogen dominance. A more holistic approach to hormonal health can yield far better results for managing menstrual irregularities or acne, without the side effects linked to contraceptives.

Hormone Replacement Therapy and Estrogen Dominance

As people age, natural declines in hormone levels cause menopause for women and andropause for men. This hormonal decline often brings various symptoms, including fatigue, irritability, night sweats, reduced libido, and increased cardiovascular risk. Hormone replacement therapy (HRT) or (TRT) aims to mitigate these symptoms by replenishing hormones, though it's often done in ways that may be detrimental.

One issue with conventional HRT is that it's frequently prescribed without testing current hormone levels. Effective Endocrinological Intervention at the most advanced level includes Bio Identical Hormone Replacement Therapy BHRT requires knowing each person's unique hormone profile, so thorough testing should include cortisol, FSH, DHEA, pregnenolone, estrogen, progesterone, and testosterone. Furthermore, the delivery method matters: creams, patches, tablets, and pellets each interact with the body differently. Pills, for instance, are processed by the liver, changing their structure and sometimes creating forms that are unnatural and possibly harmful to the body.

Bioidentical hormone replacement therapy (BHRT), where hormones are molecularly identical to those produced naturally in the body, offers a safer alternative. Unfortunately, many doctors prescribe synthetic hormones, which are altered on a molecular level to be patentable. These synthetic hormones may come with significant side effects, including heightened risks for cancer, blood clots, and heart disease.

Among bioidentical hormone delivery methods, pellets offer a particularly effective solution. Implanted under the skin, they release a steady flow of hormones throughout the day, mimicking the body's natural hormone rhythms. Pellets are associated with improved well-being in men and in some cases women, making them a superior choice compared to other HRT forms.

Please be aware that many doctors are educated by big pharma reps with their bias to prefer injectable synthetic testosterone agents at times covered by insurance, or with the misleading information that these oil esters of testosterone (cypionate, nandrolone etc) will not convert into estrogen as readily as bio identical pellets or cream. Dr Jonathan Wright, in an interview with me, calls these synthetic versions of testosterone "alien molecules" that the body will accumulate and increase the risk of infertility, cancer or heart disease.

The other challenge with using pellets or creams is that your body will no longer produce its own testosterone. This is only true to the extent the body will reduce the production by about 30% of an already poor ability to produce sufficient testosterone to thrive as an aging male or female. The difference of adding in a generous and calculated daily supply from the creams applied on the skin or the pellets slowly melting during the heat of the body during the day and less testosterone released during the night while one sleeps.

Another problem is most doctors have been using testosterone pellets with the wrong delivery system. This is concentrated in the pellets and can cause pain for days even weeks after being inserted just under the skin in the buttocks area. We only work with doctors who use the highest quality pellets concentrated to the right mg dose. Each pellet the size of a grain of rice has either 100 mg or 200 mg of bio identical testosterone.

I had two clients who both had poor experiences with the use of pellets with prior doctors until they were introduced to my network of highly trained doctors who have been doing hormone intervention for 20 to thirty years. The results were these correct protocols provided the best outcomes.

I have noticed as I am passing the age of 71, taking the right supplements to help control estrogen metabolites, herbs that release more bio available hormones exerting positive effects on the body, is critical to success in achieving the desired results to slow or reverse aging.

I believe we must take into account the body is kinda like an orchestra which requires dozens of hormones to be balanced starting with adrenal cortisol levels, estrogen, not just testosterone levels. When done properly as I am educating you to appreciate the reduction in inflammation, improvement in sexual interest, performance and muscle density, reductions in body fat, increases in energy is a game changer.

It's commonly understood that testosterone therapy in males can lead to testicular shrinkage—a physiologic response due to reduced endogenous testosterone production. As Dr. Ron Rothenberg notes, this effect is largely cosmetic and does not typically impact health or performance. For those concerned, some physicians prescribe agents like clomiphene (Clomid) or human chorionic gonadotropin (HCG) to stimulate the body's natural testosterone production. However, it's important to be aware that these interventions can carry side effects, particularly in women, including breast tenderness, nausea, dizziness, and in rare cases, an increased risk of ovarian complications.

Let's take a closer look at a unique formulation that combines four key hormones—Pregnenolone, DHEA, androgens, along with botanicals like DIM and chrysin—to help clear harmful estrogens. When blended into a single topical cream free from the toxic chemicals found in many conventional products, this solution makes it easier to optimize hormone levels to those seen in youth. I've also developed a complementary cream containing a very low dose of progesterone, paired with skin-friendly herbs designed to promote clear, healthy skin and combat acne.

While many factors can contribute to estrogen dominance, taking control of one's hormonal health through balanced weight management, considering alternatives to synthetic hormones, and working with knowledgeable healthcare providers can lead to better health outcomes and improve quality of life.

Part Three
The Delgado Protocol

In this section of the book, I lay out the exact steps to take to begin to heal your estrogen dominance: What to do first, second, third, and so on, to lose weight, reduce your risk of many cancers, improve your acne, regrow your hair, and bring your hormones back in to balance.

Chapter Seven: Detox Your Environment

The power to protect yourself lies in the choices you make every day. It's true: the xenoestrogens I discussed in the first part of this book may seem impossible to avoid, but your body is remarkably resilient and capable of bouncing back once you start making changes.

A powerful study from 2016 at UC Berkeley showed this resilience firsthand. When a group of teenage girls switched to natural cosmetics—just for three days!—they saw drastic reductions in the levels of harmful chemicals in their blood. Parabens dropped by 44%, phthalates by 27%, and triclosan by 36%. This remarkable result proves that small changes in your purchasing habits can have big impacts on your hormone health.

In this chapter, I'll walk you through the essentials for creating a safer home. I'll give you specific, actionable steps to take—so you can be confident in your ability to reduce your xenoestrogen exposure. Let's explore how to swap out harmful products for healthier options, making a big difference one small step at a time.

Out with the Old: Products to Avoid

Plastic containers, water bottles, cling wrap, and cutlery - These common items leach xenoestrogens into your food and drinks.

Styrofoam plates and cups - A major source of toxins, especially when heated.

Flame-retardant-treated fabrics and furniture - Often unlabeled, these items give off gas chemicals while you sleep.

Conventional personal care products – Say goodbye to antibacterial soaps, hand sanitizers, mainstream cosmetics, and anything with artificial fragrance.

Conventional household cleaners – Traditional cleaners, bleach, and detergents are common xenoestrogen sources.

Solvents – If you must use solvents like rubbing alcohol or paint thinners, always wear gloves to reduce exposure.

In with the New: Products to Embrace

Glass food containers and glass water bottles – Safe and stylish, these help keep xenoestrogens out of your food and drink.

Water filter – The ultimate is a reverse osmosis system, but a charcoal filter is a budget-friendly option. Even a simple filtered showerhead can make a big difference in reducing your exposure. A bigger investment would be to have a full house water purification system because when you shower or wash your hands you are exposed to an unnecessary amount of chemicals that absorb right into your body within seconds.

Natural household cleaners – Affordable brands like Seventh Generation offer effective, toxin-free options.

Natural personal care products – Look for paraben-free, phthalate-free options at your local natural grocery or mainstream stores like Target.

Your choices are powerful, and these simple swaps can have profound effects on your health. Let's dive into the specifics and give you a clear roadmap to detox your surroundings and safeguard your hormones. You're just a few choices away from creating a safer, healthier environment for yourself and those you love.

Chapter Eight: Supplements

Detoxify, Balance, and Renew: Your Next Step in the Delgado Protocol

Transforming your health begins with conscious choices—starting with what you bring into your home and body. By shifting your purchasing habits and introducing strategic supplements, you can drastically reduce your exposure to xenoestrogens and other toxic disruptors. In this critical stage of the Delgado Protocol, I'll guide you in equipping your body with the tools it needs to eliminate harmful hormones and reclaim hormonal balance.

After working with thousands of clients, I've found that meaningful symptom relief is what drives real, lasting change. That's why I recommend beginning with targeted supplements before diving into dietary changes. These supplements provide your body with essential support to begin clearing out toxic estrogens and preventing new ones from forming. Once you feel that shift—more energy, clearer skin, better mood—you'll naturally be inspired to continue your wellness journey through my customized nutrition and lifestyle plan.

While a clean, nutrient-rich diet and the lifestyle habits covered in Chapter 10 are essential, they alone may not fully resolve stubborn symptoms of estrogen dominance like acne, hair loss, or weight gain. Relying only on food often leads to slow or minimal progress, which can stall motivation. Strategic supplementation jumpstarts results, preparing your body to better respond to dietary improvements.

The Three Core Supplement Categories for Estrogen Balance

To effectively address estrogen dominance, I recommend three powerful supplement categories:

1. Estrogen Blockers

Your body produces different types of estrogen—some beneficial, others harmful. The "good" estrogen, 2OHE, supports heart health, bone strength, and fat metabolism. The "bad" estrogen, 16aOHE, is linked to hormone-related cancers, acne, and fat gain.

Key Ingredients:

DIM and I3C: Derived from cruciferous vegetables, these compounds help your body favor the production of beneficial estrogens while deactivating harmful ones. DIM (diindolylmethane), in particular, is a potent detoxifier and anti-cancer agent. While foods like broccoli and kale contain these compounds, you'd need to eat pounds of raw veggies daily to match the therapeutic dose found in supplements.

Wasabi Root Powder: A member of the Brassica family, wasabi contains highly concentrated isothiocyanates (ITCs) that activate detox enzymes in the liver, helping to neutralize and eliminate harmful estrogens more effectively than other cruciferous vegetables.

2. Liver Support

Your liver plays a central role in processing hormones and toxins. But modern environmental overload—from food, plastics, and pollution—can leave it sluggish and inefficient.

Key Ingredients:

Astragalus: This adaptogenic herb supports liver function while enhancing immunity, reducing stress, and offering anti-aging benefits.

Turmeric: A powerful antioxidant and anti-inflammatory, turmeric protects the liver, supports detoxification, and helps prevent the conversion of testosterone to estrogen.

Silymarin (Milk Thistle Extract): Renowned for regenerating liver cells and protecting against oxidative stress, silymarin enhances your liver's capacity to clear excess estrogen.

---

3. Methyl Donors

These nutrients help safely remove excess estrogen by aiding in methylation—a biochemical process crucial for detox.

Key Ingredients:

DMG, TMG, MSM, B12, and 5-MTHF: These compounds support estrogen elimination and are key components in our *Hair Skin Detox* formula, which complements *EstroBlock* through all three phases of estrogen metabolism.

Introducing Estroblock Vitality: Cellular Health, Hormonal Balance & Anti-Aging in One

Estroblock Vitality is the next evolution in hormonal and cellular health. Formulated with 15 science-backed ingredients, it supports detoxification, hormone balance, skin health, and cognitive function—all while promoting graceful aging.

Highlights of *Estroblock Vitality*:

Cellular Renewal with Spermidine: Encourages autophagy, your body's natural process of cleaning and rejuvenating cells.

Detox Enhancement with Calcium D-Glucarate: Assists in the safe removal of hormones and toxins.

Antioxidant Protection from Sulforaphane: Activates the NRF2 pathway, stimulating your body's natural antioxidant defenses.

Hormonal Harmony from I3C: Supports healthy estrogen metabolism.

Restorative Sleep & Joint Support from Niacinamide (B3): Promotes better rest and improved mobility.

Skin Radiance from Apigenin: Soothes and revitalizes your complexion.

Brain & Heart Health from Spermidine: Supports cognition, memory, immune strength, and cardiovascular vitality.

Pure, Potent, and Clean

Estroblock Vitality is free of gluten, soy, dairy, shellfish, fish, and common allergens. It's vegan, non-GMO, and designed for those who demand the highest quality for their body and mind.

Start Your Transformation

With these carefully formulated supplements, you'll begin to feel lighter, more energized, and hormonally balanced—setting the stage for deeper transformations through diet and lifestyle. This is your moment to take control, feel amazing, and embrace your journey to optimal health.

Chapter Nine:
Diet

Transforming Health with the Delgado Protocol: A Personal Journey

When my dad was in his seventies, he was like many older American men—dependent on medications for blood pressure and diabetes. I offered to help him through nutrition and lifestyle changes but his wife, like many, followed conventional medical advice: avoid starches, increase meat and dairy. My recommendation—foods like potatoes, beans, and brown rice—seemed too radical at the time.

Fast forward nearly fifteen years. At 83, he began showing signs of memory loss and early Alzheimer's. This time, he and his wife were ready to listen. I transitioned him to a whole-food, plant-based diet, cut out oils and refined sugars, and implemented a gentle exercise plan. Too weak to train, he stood on a whole-body vibration platform while Tesla Max AC current electrodes stimulated his muscles.

Within three weeks, his blood pressure normalized, his medications were discontinued, and he began taking targeted supplements and bioidentical hormones. Remarkably, his diabetes and Alzheimer's symptoms reversed. He became himself again—joyful, engaged, cracking jokes that made us all laugh.

The Heart of the Delgado Protocol: Healthy, Not Hungry

This isn't a restrictive diet—it's about abundance. You can eat to satisfaction with nutrient-dense, fiber-rich, plant-based foods. The key? Eating in sequence: start with the lowest calorie, most nutrient-packed foods like greens and fruits, then gradually move to heartier fare like sweet potatoes, beans, and whole grains.

For weight loss, we recommend following Dr. Valter Longo's advice: reduce body fat gradually—about ½ to 1 pound per week—especially after age 65. To gain or sustain weight, reverse the sequence: begin with calorie-dense whole plant foods like nuts, seeds, avocados, and grains, then finish with vegetables and fruits.

This is intuitive eating—no counting calories or feeling deprived. It's about flooding your body with healing nutrients.

The Power of Nutrient Density

Take Chef Shayda, for example. She once followed a restrictive diet prescribed by a metabolic doctor—it didn't work. Then she met Dr. Joel Fuhrman, who emphasized plant-based nutrient density. She lost over 120 pounds and has kept it off for 17 years by embracing food sequencing and whole plant foods.

Science backs this approach. Whole, plant-based diets provide every essential nutrient—including protein—and are naturally anti-inflammatory.

Protein Myths—Busted

There's no shortage of protein on this plan. Here are some star sources:

Pumpkin seeds: 32g per cup

Lentils: 18g

Edamame: 17g

Black beans: 15g

Even sweet potatoes, spinach, quinoa, and broccoli contribute to your daily protein intake. The World Health Organization states a 155-pound adult needs only 35 grams of protein daily. Athletes or larger individuals might need up to 60 grams.

Most of my clients consume 45 to 80 grams of highly absorbable plant protein daily—more than enough to support muscle growth, healing, and vitality.

Mike Mentzer, Mr. Universe and heavyweight winner of Mr. Olympia 1979, said gaining muscle requires only a modest increase in protein—about 6 extra grams per day for sustained growth. With consistency, genetics, and hormone optimization, a man could double his lean muscle mass over five years.

Healthy Fats—Not Oils

Fat is essential—but only in its whole form. The Delgado Protocol includes fats from olives, seeds, nuts, chia, and avocados. We avoid processed oils, which cause red blood cells to clump together, reducing oxygen delivery throughout the body. This impairs energy and contributes to chronic disease.

I've analyzed thousands of blood samples under a microscope. One tablespoon of oil can visibly reduce blood cell flexibility. Our smallest capillaries are 7 microns wide—yet red blood cells are 9 microns. They must fold to pass through. When clumped together by oils, they can't. This creates fatigue, poor circulation, and increased disease risk.

Our protocol emphasizes omega-3-rich foods and minimizes omega-6 and omega-9 fats, restoring a healthy balance critical to preventing cancer, heart disease, and diabetes.

Whole Foods Only

Packaged foods are often loaded with xenoestrogens, oils, and refined sugar. Whole foods, by contrast, provide antioxidants, fiber, and natural compounds that promote detoxification and longevity.

A Day on the Delgado Protocol

Here's a sample day to inspire you:

Breakfast:

Bananas, strawberries, blueberries, soaked walnuts, Brazil nuts, hemp, chia, and flax seeds, with cold-pressed beet or green juice.

Lunch:

Raw Thai mango salad with carrot ginger soup.

Snack:

Carrots and celery with hummus, a handful of olives.

Dinner:

Sweet potato burger over greens with broccoli salad.

Sweet Potato Burger Recipe:

2 cans white beans, mashed

1 large cooked sweet potato

2 tbsp tahini

1 tsp Cajun seasoning

¼ cup gluten-free flour

2 tsp coconut nectar

Gluten-free breadcrumbs

1 tbsp vegetable broth

Salt & pepper

Mix all ingredients, shape into patties, coat with breadcrumbs, and cook in broth until golden on both sides.

Chapter Ten: Lifestyle changes

Beyond the Physical: A Holistic Guide to Longevity and Vitality

Living a vibrant, extended life requires more than just eating well or maintaining a skincare routine. True longevity is achieved through a full-spectrum approach that includes physical, mental, and emotional health. This guide explores the critical pillars of wellness: stress regulation, restorative sleep, mindful movement, detoxification, optimal nutrition, and purposeful mindset.

Rethinking Energy and Stress

Modern life often drives us toward quick fixes like caffeine and sugar to power through fatigue. These stimulants overwork the adrenal glands and thyroid, disrupting hormonal balance and fueling a cycle of dependency. As cortisol levels drop, thyroid hormones become less effective, resulting in burnout and chronic fatigue—even when standard blood tests appear normal.

More accurate insight often comes from saliva or urine tests that track daily hormone rhythms. Addressing adrenal fatigue involves reducing stimulant use and incorporating adaptogens and supportive nutrients like iodine and glandular extracts.. Replacing caffeine with paraxanthine—a cleaner metabolite of caffeine—can provide smoother energy without taxing the adrenals.

Mental Clarity and Guided Relaxation

The nervous system benefits greatly from daily stress-reduction practices. Guided imagery, theta-wave meditation, and sound therapy help reset your emotional baseline. Just a few minutes of focused relaxation, particularly in the morning and before bed, can recalibrate your stress response. Tools like those found at *7pillarscoaching.com* are designed to enhance adrenal and thyroid health through mental conditioning.

Reclaiming Sleep for Repair

Vital hormonal activity peaks between 8 p.m. and 5 a.m., making early sleep essential. Staying up late or using stimulants disturbs the body's ability to heal, regenerate, and regulate hormones. Deep, consistent sleep patterns have been linked to longer lifespan, improved cognitive performance, and lower disease risk.

Exercise as Detox and Hormonal Balance

Movement drives detoxification and hormonal harmony. Sweating eliminates toxins and helps regulate estrogen. While extended high-intensity exercise can suppress testosterone and shift hormonal ratios, shorter, strategic workouts are more beneficial. A balanced regimen might include:

Two 12-minute high-intensity sessions per week

One session of yoga or tai chi

Two flow-state workouts at a conversational pace with a heart rate between 110-135 bpm

Mastering the Mind

Mental programming shapes physical outcomes. Limiting beliefs and chronic stress sabotage progress. Techniques like NLP (Neuro-Linguistic Programming), Time Line Therapy, and trans phenomena guide the subconscious to adopt empowering patterns. Scripts like those available through *foreveryoungevent.com* support inner transformation:

"With every breath, I am grounded. I invite clarity and peace into my day. I awaken with strength and joy."

In these guided sessions, we rewire patterns, enhance decision-making, and attract positive mentorship and connection. Mental training creates the foundation for sustainable habits and improved health outcomes.

The Real Causes Behind Chronic Disease

The surge in heart disease, cancer, and diabetes is often blamed on aging, but lifestyle and environmental toxins play a far greater role. Processed foods, industrial chemicals, and endocrine disruptors—such as PCBs and pesticides—interfere with hormonal function and cellular repair.

Detox as a Daily Practice

The body's detox systems thrive on nutrient density and minimal toxin exposure. Supporting detoxification involves:

High-fiber, plant-based meals

Hydration with purified water

Intermittent fasting

Supplements like milk thistle, glutathione, and activated charcoal

Infrared saunas and consistent sweating

Reducing chemical exposure by choosing organic foods and clean personal care products is equally important. Stress management amplifies detox effectiveness by reducing internal toxin production.

The Nutrient Foundation

A robust immune system and cellular resilience rely on whole foods and strategic supplementation. Key nutrients include:

Antioxidants: Vitamin C, E, selenium

Essential fats: Plant-based omega-3s

Gut health agents: Probiotics, prebiotics

Energy cofactors: B vitamins, magnesium, zinc

Phytonutrients: Found in colorful fruits and vegetables

Meal timing also matters—intermittent fasting enhances insulin sensitivity and supports cellular repair.

Exercise for Oxygen and Vitality

Regular physical activity improves oxygenation, strengthens immunity, and lowers inflammation. Resistance training preserves lean muscle, while aerobic movement supports cardiovascular health. Personalized programs aid in recovery and longevity, even for individuals facing chronic conditions.

The Role of Connection and Rest

Strong social bonds and emotional intimacy boost immune function and reduce disease risk. Communities known for longevity share common traits: close relationships, shared meals, and daily physical activity. Sleep, too, plays a vital role. Practices that enhance rest include limiting screen time, creating calming evening rituals, and using herbal supports like chamomile or valerian root.

Blood Microscopy: Your Inner Health Mirror

Live and dry blood analysis reveals nutrient status, oxidative stress, and inflammation. Processed oils and fats can visibly impair oxygen transport in blood. Real-time improvements from dietary shifts underscore the body's responsiveness to lifestyle changes.

Plant-Based Nutrition for Prevention

Diets rich in greens, beans, onions, mushrooms, berries, and seeds—popularized by Dr. Joel Fuhrman as G-BOMBS—offer powerful protection against disease. These foods detoxify the body, strengthen immunity, and fight inflammation. Intermittent fasting, juicing, and incorporating foods rich in polyphenols (like green tea and turmeric) support cellular repair.

Legacy of Pioneers in Health

Dr. Dean Ornish proved lifestyle medicine can reverse heart disease through plant-based diets and emotional wellness.

Dr. Ernest Wynder linked dietary fat to cancer risk and advocated for community-supported wellness.

Dr. Meyer Friedman demonstrated the vascular damage caused by dietary oils and championed nutrient-dense, personalized care.

Suzanne Somers promoted bioidentical hormone therapies and holistic living for vitality, yet she consumed far too much animal product ignoring the fact that chicken and fish have as much cholesterol as red meat. even though your body produces all the cholesterol you need. When you consume cholesterol and fatty animal-based products, triglycerides increase. That combination leads to dangerously high risk of cancer diabetes, high blood pressure and heart disease not to mention obesity, which further worsens your chance of premature death!

Emerging Therapies and Innovation

New approaches like peptide therapy, hyperbaric oxygen, cryotherapy, and cyclic variations in adaptive conditioning-CVAC are expanding the potential to treat chronic illness and enhance vitality. These tools, when integrated with foundational wellness practices, deliver powerful synergistic effects.

A Deeper Look at Hormonal Imbalance

Hormone-disrupting chemicals are everywhere—from plastics to water supplies. Estrogen dominance contributes to reproductive disorders, early puberty, and hormone-sensitive cancers. Reducing exposure and supporting the body's ability to detoxify these compounds is crucial.

Exposing the Food-Pharma Feedback Loop

The collusion between food and pharmaceutical industries perpetuates illness. Companies profit from both harmful food products and the medications designed to treat the resulting conditions. Tackling this requires systemic reform and greater transparency, and informed consumer choices.

The Way Forward

We each have the power to break the cycle of poor health. Start with daily habits:

Shift to a whole-food, plant-based diet

Support detox through movement, fasting, and supplementation

Prioritize deep sleep and mental clarity

Build meaningful relationships

Educate yourself and others

Join wellness initiatives like the ForeverYoungevent.com and explore deeper insights in "Stop Aging Now", Peptides and the simple methods revealed in this to overcome a society poisioned by Estrogen Dominance.

Together, we can reclaim health—not just for ourselves, but for generations to come. The path begins with awareness and the commitment to consistent, empowered choices. The future of wellness is not prescribed—it is cultivated.

Part 4 Introduction To Peptides

Nick Delgado, PhD, ABAAHP,

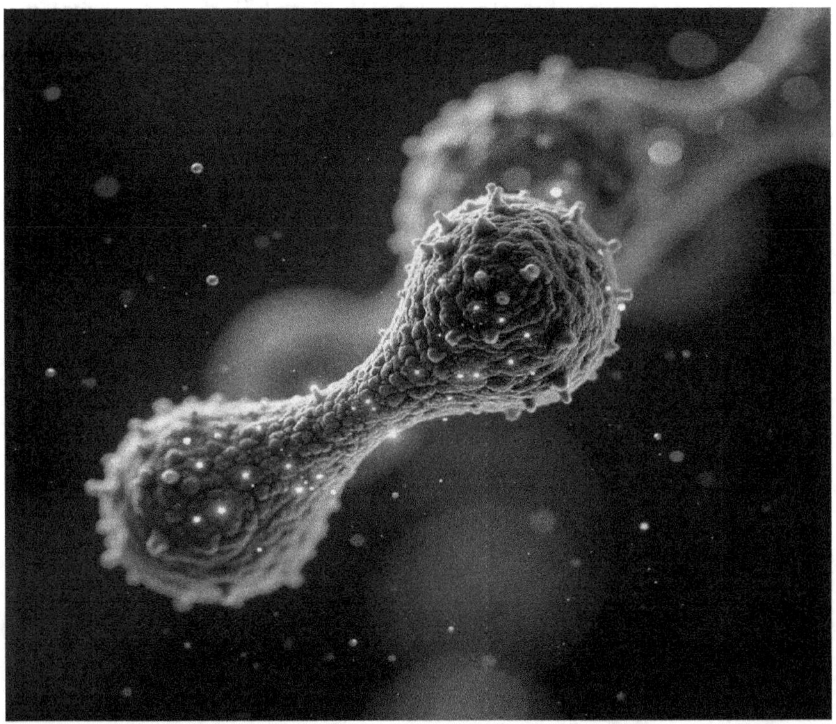

In my book Stop Aging Now I shared the 7 pillars and secrets to get in great shape. In the first section we discussed the importance of managing estrogen dominance that affects men and women in each stage of our lives.

The idea that short chain natural amino acids called peptides can modulate and improve the balance of virtually hundreds of hormones to achieve ideal health is shared in this section.

Welcome to the *How to Lose Weight Effortlessly Section 2 Peptides* – a comprehensive exploration into one of the most exciting and transformative fields in modern health and medicine.

Peptides, once reserved for specialized clinical settings, have rapidly evolved into powerful tools for healing, performance optimization, anti-aging, and overall human enhancement. Acting as precise biological messengers, peptides regulate vital functions such as tissue repair, hormone balance, cognitive function, immune resilience, fat metabolism, and cellular rejuvenation.

Their specificity and versatility position them at the forefront of regenerative and personalized medicine.

This section is designed for health enthusiasts, and individuals seeking to unlock the full potential of their bodies and minds. It provides both foundational knowledge and advanced insights into the science, application, and future of peptide therapy.

I got an urgent health education call a few months ago. There was a construction accident. The man said he was hurt badly without any hope.

"I have practically no pain at this point, it actually feels like a miracle. My foot still has a lot of swelling, but pretty much no resting pain. I haven't attempted to put much pressure on it yet. I have an appointment with a Podiatrist next week for X Rays and to see what's currently going on. Feels just like nerve stuff at this point."

I have family in Hawaii in their 70's and they are inquiring about the peptides. I was just talking about you, can I refer someone to talk to you?"

Darryl Herndon

Across the segments ahead, you will discover:

- **The science behind peptides** and how they support regenerative processes at the cellular level
- **The difference between oral and injectable peptides**, including usage guidelines for each
- **Protocol designs** tailored to fat loss, recovery, cognition, muscle growth, and longevity
- **Case studies** demonstrating real-world transformations using personalized peptide stacks
- **Expert perspectives** from clinical leaders like Dr. Nick Delgado, Iman Barr MD, Maryanne Hannaney MD, James LaVelle, RPh, and Dr. Andrew Huberman, Edwin Lee MD, endocrinologist, Michael Grossman MD and William Seeds MD
- **Emerging trends**, including gene editing, smart peptides, AI-driven personalized therapy, and ethical considerations for the future of enhancement medicine
-

At **Delgado Protocol for Health and Delgadolabs.com**, we believe peptides represent more than just a new therapeutic category—they represent a paradigm shift in how we define health, longevity, and human potential.

Now is the time to embrace the next evolution of medicine.

Welcome to the future. Welcome to How to lose weight effortlessly utilizing peptides.

Segment one Introduction to Peptides

- The role of peptides in biology and medicine
- Peptides vs traditional drugs: precision and safety
- Regenerative, hormonal, cognitive, and anti-aging applications

Segment 2 Oral Peptides (Simplified Guide and Deep Dive)

- Advantages of oral delivery
- Key oral peptides: BPC-157, MK-677, Dihexa, Epitalon
- Stacking strategies and lifestyle integration

Segment 3 Injectable Peptides (Expanded Guide)

- Bioavailability advantages of injectables
- Detailed research protocols for BPC-157, TB-500, CJC-1295, Ipamorelin, Semaglutide
- Smart stacking for fat loss, recovery, and growth

Segment 4: Additional Peptides (For Educational Purposes Only)

- Selank, Semax, Thymosin Alpha-1, GHK-Cu, DSIP, Tesamorelin
- Emerging clinical uses and experimental protocols

Segment 5: Expert Insights from the Delgado Video Channel

- Recovery, brain health, and real-world case outcomes

Segment 6: Building Your Personalized Peptide Protocol

- How to set goals, select peptides, dose properly, cycle wisely, and monitor progress
- Fat loss, cognitive optimization, injury recovery, and anti-aging frameworks

Segment 7: Advanced Peptide Protocols and Case Studies

- Recovery after surgery or injury
- Hormonal rejuvenation for athletes
- Cognitive repair and enhancement strategies
- Metabolic resets for fat loss and insulin control

Segment 8: Advanced Applications and Future Directions of Peptide Therapy

- Regenerative medicine, neuroprotection, anti-aging interventions
- Personalized medicine and AI-driven therapy customization
- Combining peptides with exosomes, stem cells, and genetic medicine

Segment 9: The Future of Peptide Therapy and Emerging Applications

- Gene editing and peptide-assisted gene therapy
- New peptides for cognitive resilience and chronic disease management
- Global health applications and low-resource medical innovation

Segment 10: The Future of Peptide Therapy — Unlocking Human Potential

- Smart peptides, dynamic dosing, and AI-enhanced health optimization
- Ethical considerations in enhancement medicine
- Redefining aging, recovery, resilience, and peak human performance

Segment One: Introduction to Peptides

Peptides are small chains of amino acids that are essential to the body's functions. While proteins are larger chains of amino acids, peptides serve a similar purpose—they act as molecular messengers that regulate vital biological functions. The natural occurrence and synthesis of peptides in the body make them an important part of many physiological processes. These chains of amino acids trigger specific biological reactions in cells, tissues, and organs, playing roles in processes ranging from tissue repair and immune function to hormone regulation and metabolism.

A peptide's effectiveness lies in its specificity. Unlike traditional medications, which can often have broad and sometimes harmful side effects, peptides can be designed to target specific tissues or organs in the body, ensuring that their effects are precise and localized. This characteristic makes them highly effective for regenerative medicine, where the goal is to accelerate the body's natural healing processes rather than suppress symptoms.

The concept of peptide therapy emerged with the realization that peptides could act as natural enhancers of the body's own regenerative processes. For instance, peptides like BPC-157 and TB-500 are used for accelerated tissue repair, helping to heal injuries and reduce inflammation.

Others, such as MK-677 and CJC-1295, are used to stimulate the body's production of growth hormone, which can improve fat metabolism, increase muscle retention, and support healthy aging.

At Delgado Labs, we recognize the immense value peptides offer in the realm of wellness and medicine. Through both oral and injectable peptides, we offer a comprehensive range of products tailored to meet individual health goals.

Whether you're looking to recover from an injury, improve sleep quality, enhance cognitive performance, or slow the aging process, peptides offer a highly customizable and effective solution.

This Section introduces the foundational concepts behind peptides, including their definition, the science of how they work in the body, and the potential benefits they offer for specific health conditions. We will also delve into the importance of choosing the right peptides, their modes of administration, and the growing role they play in modern medicine.

Peptide therapy is gaining traction across multiple fields of health, it's important to understand how they function, their therapeutic applications, and their impact on health optimization.

The Science Behind Peptides Peptides are composed of amino acids, which are the building blocks of proteins. These amino acids are linked together by peptide bonds. Unlike proteins, which are long chains of hundreds of amino acids, peptides are shorter, usually containing fewer than 50 amino acids. The unique sequence of amino acids in each peptide determines its function in the body.

When peptides are synthesized in the body, they act as signaling molecules. They are involved in a variety of physiological processes, including cellular communication, immune function, metabolism, and tissue repair.

For example, some peptides function by binding to specific receptors on the surface of cells, initiating a cascade of biochemical reactions that result in the desired physiological response.

One of the key features of peptides is their ability to interact with specific receptors on target cells. This makes them much more precise than many traditional drugs, which often interact with multiple systems in the body, sometimes causing unwanted side effects. Peptides, on the other hand, can be engineered to target specific receptors, resulting in a more efficient and safer therapeutic effect.

Peptides in **Regenerative Medicine** is one of the most significant applications of peptides in medicine is in regenerative therapies. Regenerative medicine focuses on harnessing the body's own healing mechanisms to repair or replace damaged tissues. Peptides play a crucial role in this process by stimulating tissue regeneration and accelerating healing.

For example, BPC-157, often referred to as a "healing peptide," has been shown to accelerate the healing of muscles, tendons, and ligaments. By promoting angiogenesis (the formation of new blood vessels) and increasing collagen production, BPC-157 speeds up the recovery process for injuries. Similarly, TB-500, another peptide, has been found to enhance cell migration and promote tissue regeneration, making it a valuable tool for athletes and anyone recovering from injury or surgery.

Another key peptide in regenerative medicine is Thymosin Beta-4, which is involved in tissue repair and wound healing. This peptide has shown promise in repairing damaged tissues in the cardiovascular system, helping to regenerate endothelial cells and promote new blood vessel growth. Its regenerative effects are not limited to soft tissues; Thymosin Beta-4 has also demonstrated potential in improving bone healing.

Peptide Therapy for hormone regulation is yet another area where peptides are proving to be highly effective. As we age, our bodies experience a decline in natural hormone production, which can lead to symptoms like fatigue, muscle loss, increased body fat, and cognitive decline. Peptide therapy can help restore the balance of hormones by stimulating the body's natural hormone production.

Peptides like CJC-1295, Ipamorelin, and MK-677 are used to stimulate the release of growth hormone from the pituitary gland. **Growth hormone** plays a critical role in regulating metabolism, promoting muscle growth, and maintaining youthful skin and energy levels.

As people age, their growth hormone levels naturally decline, leading to symptoms of aging. By using peptides to stimulate the production of growth hormone, individuals can reverse some of these symptoms and improve overall vitality.

For those with **testosterone** deficiency, peptides like Gonadorelin (GnRH) can be used to stimulate the production of testosterone in men. This peptide is often used in hormone replacement therapy (HRT) protocols to restore testosterone levels and alleviate symptoms like low libido, fatigue, and muscle loss.

Peptides for Cognitive Enhancement Cognitive health is an area where peptides are gaining significant attention, particularly as more people seek ways to enhance brain function and prevent age-related cognitive decline. Peptides like Dihexa, Semax, and Noopept are being studied for their potential to improve memory, learning, and overall brain function.

Dihexa, for instance, has been shown to promote neurogenesis, the growth of new neurons, and improve synaptic plasticity, which is the ability of the brain to form new connections between neurons. This makes Dihexa an exciting prospect for individuals looking to improve **cognitive** performance or recover from traumatic brain injuries.

Semax, another cognitive peptide, increases levels of brain-derived neurotrophic factor (BDNF), a protein that supports the growth, survival, and differentiation of neurons. Semax has been found to enhance memory, attention, and overall cognitive function, particularly in individuals with neurodegenerative conditions like Alzheimer's.

Peptides for Fat Loss and Metabolism

Fat loss and metabolic health are two areas where peptides are making a big impact. Peptides like AOD-9604 and Semaglutide have been shown to stimulate fat breakdown and improve insulin sensitivity, making them useful tools for individuals struggling with weight management or metabolic disorders.

AOD-9604 is a peptide fragment derived from human growth hormone that specifically targets fat cells. It has been shown to stimulate lipolysis (the breakdown of fat) without affecting blood glucose levels, making it an ideal choice for targeted fat loss. Semaglutide, a **GLP-1** agonist, works by regulating appetite and improving insulin sensitivity, making it effective for weight loss and blood sugar control. I prefer the newer GLP-2 and GLP-3.

Peptide Therapy for Anti-Aging Anti-aging is one of the most popular applications of peptide therapy, as peptides have the ability to slow down the aging process at the cellular level.

Peptides like Epitalon and GHK-Cu have shown promise in promoting cellular regeneration, enhancing skin elasticity, and even extending lifespan by repairing DNA and protecting telomeres.

Epithalon, in particular, has been studied for its ability to activate telomerase, an enzyme that helps maintain the length of telomeres—the protective caps at the end of chromosomes.

As we age, our telomeres naturally shorten, which leads to cellular aging and a decline in tissue function. By stimulating telomerase production, Epitalon helps prevent telomere shortening, thus promoting **longevity** and slowing down the aging process.

GHK-Cu is another peptide with strong anti-aging properties. It has been shown to stimulate collagen production, improve skin regeneration, and reduce wrinkles, making it a popular choice for cosmetic anti-aging protocols. Beyond its skin benefits, GHK-Cu also has systemic effects, including enhancing tissue repair and reducing inflammation.

Peptides are becoming an essential tool in modern medicine, offering a wide range of therapeutic applications. From accelerating recovery and improving hormone balance to enhancing cognitive function and promoting longevity, peptides are proving to be versatile and effective. Their precision and ability to target specific tissues make them a powerful tool in the fight against chronic diseases, aging, and injury.

At Delgado Labs, we specialize in supporting the research for both oral and injectable peptides, offering a comprehensive range of education products to support health optimization. See courses at foreveryoungevent.com

Whether you are an athlete looking to enhance performance, an aging individual seeking to improve vitality, or someone recovering from injury, peptides offer a tailored solution to meet your unique health goals. Delgadolabs.com

Segment Two: Oral Peptides (Simplified Guide and Deep Dive)

Oral peptides have emerged as a convenient and non-invasive method for accessing the regenerative power of peptide therapy. As the field of regenerative and functional medicine continues to expand, peptides are gaining recognition as powerful tools for enhancing healing, hormonal balance, metabolic efficiency, immune function, and cognitive clarity.

Oral delivery offers a practical alternative to injections, particularly for those who seek ease, comfort, and consistency in their health regimen.

Unlike injectable peptides, which often require medical supervision, sterile technique, and careful dosing, **oral peptides** come in the form of capsules, tablets, sublingual drops, or powders—making them far more accessible for daily use. While traditional concerns about peptide degradation in the digestive tract once limited their efficacy, modern delivery systems have significantly improved bioavailability. Technologies such as enteric coatings, liposomal delivery, and enzyme inhibitors now allow many oral peptides to survive the digestive process and reach systemic circulation with measurable therapeutic effect.

Oral peptides can target a wide array of physiological goals. For instance, compounds like BPC-157 and GHK-Cu support tissue repair and inflammation control, while others like Dihexa and Noopept are designed to enhance memory, focus, and neuroplasticity.

Additionally, oral growth hormone secretagogues such as MK-677 help increase endogenous (Hormone produced naturally within the body) growth hormone production, supporting fat loss, muscle retention, and anti-aging outcomes.

The key to success with oral peptides lies in strategic use—selecting the right compounds for the right goals, maintaining consistent dosing, and understanding that benefits often accumulate over time.

When integrated into a comprehensive lifestyle that includes proper nutrition, sleep, exercise, and stress management, oral peptides can play a significant role in optimizing well-being.

This chapter provides a foundational understanding of how oral peptides work, how to use them effectively, and when they might be preferable to injectable options.

Understanding Oral Peptides

Peptides are short chains of amino acids, the fundamental building blocks of proteins, that play crucial roles in cell signaling within the body. These molecules act as messengers, telling cells how to function, repair, and maintain balance. When used as part of a therapeutic regimen, peptides can help stimulate a range of processes, from tissue repair to hormone regulation.

Oral peptides are similar in function to injectable peptides, but they must be specially formulated to endure the digestive process. The human digestive system is equipped with powerful enzymes and acidic environments that can break down peptides before they have the chance to enter the bloodstream.

To address this challenge, modern formulations incorporate protective coatings, enzyme inhibitors, and absorption-enhancing agents that allow peptides to remain intact during digestion and absorption.

For an oral peptide to be effective, it must first survive the harsh environment of the gastrointestinal (GI) tract. Once absorbed into the bloodstream, it can then trigger a specific biological effect, depending on the peptide. Some peptides work locally in the digestive system, while others provide systemic benefits, circulating throughout the body to deliver their healing effects.

The Mechanisms of Oral Peptides

Each oral peptide has its own specific mechanism of action. These actions are typically aligned with the body's natural processes, which allows peptides to work synergistically with the body's signaling systems. Below are several key mechanisms of action for popular oral peptides:

- **BPC-157**: (Body Protection Compound) This peptide is known for promoting angiogenesis, or the formation of new blood vessels. It also has potent anti-inflammatory properties that help with tissue healing and repair. Commonly used for soft tissue injuries, gut health, and inflammatory conditions, BPC-157 can reduce healing times and improve overall recovery.

- **MK-677 (Ibutamoren)**: MK-677 mimics the action of ghrelin, a hormone that stimulates the release of growth hormone (GH). By increasing growth hormone and insulin-like growth factor 1 (IGF-1), MK-677 supports muscle growth, fat loss, and improves sleep quality. It is also used for anti-aging purposes, as these hormones play significant roles in cellular repair and maintenance.
- **Dihexa**: This peptide is highly valued for its neurogenic effects, promoting the growth of brain-derived neurotrophic factor (BDNF), a protein that enhances synaptic plasticity and cognitive function. Dihexa is often used for cognitive enhancement, memory improvement, and neuroprotection, making it a powerful tool for individuals looking to boost mental clarity and learning ability.
- **Epitalon**: Epitalon has a remarkable ability to stimulate telomerase, the enzyme responsible for maintaining and repairing the protective caps at the ends of chromosomes (telomeres). This function has made Epitalon popular in anti-aging circles, as it can help reduce the effects of aging by promoting DNA repair and supporting cellular longevity. Additionally, Epitalon improves melatonin production, which aids in the regulation of sleep patterns and circadian rhythms.

Each peptide has been designed to target specific processes in the body, and their effects are generally highly specific and effective with minimal side effects. However, the response to oral peptides can vary based on individual factors like metabolism, age, and underlying health conditions.

Advantages of Oral Peptides

One of the most attractive features of oral peptides is their ease of use. Unlike injectable peptides, which require sterile preparation, syringes, and specific techniques for administration, oral peptides can be taken simply by swallowing a pill or capsule. Here are several key advantages:

- **Ease of Use**: Oral peptides are extremely user-friendly. They can be taken with or without food, making them convenient for daily use. There's no need for special training or equipment, and they can be incorporated seamlessly into your daily routine.
- **Needle-Free**: Many people are intimidated or uncomfortable with injections. Oral peptides offer a painless alternative, making them a popular choice for those seeking to avoid needles.
- **Travel-Friendly**: Since oral peptides do not require refrigeration or sterile equipment, they are easy to transport. You can take them with you on trips without worrying about refrigeration or maintaining a sterile environment.
- **Improved Compliance**: Oral peptides tend to have better user compliance, particularly for individuals who are new to peptide therapy or who find injections inconvenient. The simplicity of taking a pill encourages consistent use, which is crucial for seeing long-term benefits.

Featured Oral Peptides

Here's a closer look at some of the most popular oral peptides available and their therapeutic uses:

BPC-157 Oral

- **Best For**: Gut health, soft tissue healing, systemic inflammation
- **I have used the Dosage**: 250–500 mcg daily on an empty stomach
- **Cycling**: 4 weeks on, 1–2 weeks off
- **Tip**: Combine with collagen and vitamin C for enhanced healing

TB-500 Oral

Best For: Muscle recovery, joint health, chronic inflammation

- **Dosage**: 500–1000 mcg daily
- **Cycling**: 4–6 weeks, taken 5 days a week and 2 weeks off
- **Tip**: Works synergistically with BPC-157 for full-body repair

MK-677 Oral

- **Best For**: Muscle growth, fat loss, sleep, and recovery
- **Dosage**: 10–25 mg nightly and before love making
- **Cycling**: 8–12 weeks on, 2–4 weeks off
- **Tip**: Start at lower doses if appetite increase is too strong

Epitalon Oral or nasal spray or inject

- **Best For**: Anti-aging, deep sleep, DNA repair
- **Dosage**: 5–10 mg in the evening

- **Cycling**: 20 days on, 10 days off (use once ot twice a year)
- **Tip**: Supports melatonin production and circadian rhythms

Dihexa

1. **Best For**: Cognitive enhancement, learning, neuroprotection
2. **Dosage**: 5–10 mg in the morning.
3. **Cycling**: 4–6 weeks on, 1 week off
4. **Tip**: Combine with DHA or Alpha-GPC for amplified brain benefits
5. Injectable Peptides can work within days. For this and many other reasons we advocate doing microdosing when using injectable Peptides.
6. The easiest way to do **microdosing** is to fill up the vial of peptide powder to the top of the vial with bacteriostatic water. Then use little as possible starting in sensitive individuals with less than .10 units which is 5 units on the insulin syringe needle.
7. Then after 2 weeks gradually increase the amount to 10 units and not much above 20 units. When using too high a dose many report feeling nausea which goes away.

Oral Peptide Stacking Strategies

Stacking refers to combining two or more peptides to target multiple pathways simultaneously. This approach is particularly effective for those looking to optimize results across different health goals. Here are some recommended stacking strategies:

1. **Gut + Joint Repair**: BPC-157 + TB-500

2. These peptides can work together to accelerate healing, particularly for individuals with chronic joint pain, soft tissue injuries, or digestive issues.
3. **Sleep + Growth**: MK-677 + Epitalon A combination of MK-677 and Epitalon can enhance deep sleep while supporting growth hormone production and anti-aging processes.
4. **Neurogenesis**: Dihexa + Epitalon
5. For cognitive enhancement and longevity, stacking Dihexa and Epitalon supports brain health and cellular repair.

When stacking peptides, (using different peptides at the same time) it's important to start with low doses and assess tolerance before gradually increasing dosages. Stagger the introduction of each peptide and monitor for any adverse reactions. Using a journal or mobile app to track your progress can also help identify what works best for you. Repeat these words "My Body My Research."

Individualization Based on Age, Gender, and Goals

The effectiveness of oral peptides can vary based on an individual's age, gender, and specific health goals. For instance:

- **Younger Users**: Younger individuals often benefit most from peptides that support peak physical performance, such as Dihexa and TB-500, which promote cognitive function and recovery.
- **Older Adults**: As people age, peptides like MK-677 and Epitalon can be particularly beneficial. MK-677 supports lean muscle mass and recovery, while Epitalon works to reduce the effects of aging by supporting cellular repair and maintaining telomere length.

- **Gender Considerations**: Women may prefer protocols that are less intense and involve longer rest periods between cycles. Hormonal fluctuations can make women more sensitive to certain peptides, particularly those that influence growth hormone or insulin-like growth factor.

Before starting any peptide regimen, it's crucial to consult with a healthcare professional familiar with peptide therapy, especially if you are combining peptides with hormone therapy or prescription medications. Oral Peptides may take several days or weeks to experience improvements.

Oral peptides can be very potent and it's best to take them separate from the time you are using injectable peptides.

Lifestyle Integration and Clinical Observations

At Delgado Protocol, we have seen great success when oral peptides are used as part of a comprehensive health regimen. The inclusion of lifestyle factors such as plant-based nutrition, resistance training, high-quality sleep, and stress management can significantly enhance the effects of peptides. Here are some examples from our practice:

- **BPC-157**: Clients using BPC-157 for gut healing have reported not only improved digestion but also better skin health, increased energy, and enhanced mood.
- **MK-677**: This peptide has helped older adults build lean muscle mass and recover from workouts more effectively, even when they previously struggled with post-exercise recovery.
- **Dihexa**: Users of Dihexa have noticed noticeable improvements in memory retention and cognitive function within just three weeks of use.

These clinical outcomes align with existing research and further support the efficacy of oral peptides as part of a broader approach to health and wellness.

Tracking Results and Avoiding Pitfalls

When using oral peptides, it's crucial to track progress to ensure optimal results:

- **Start Low and Go Slow**: Begin with lower doses to assess tolerance, especially with peptides like MK-677 and Dihexa, which can cause appetite changes or other side effects.
- **Avoid Overuse**: Peptides work best when used cyclically. Overuse can reduce their effectiveness and lead to receptor desensitization.
- **Track Results**: Use a tracking system to monitor changes in symptoms, energy, sleep quality, cognitive performance, and physical recovery. Periodic assessments, such as blood tests or feedback from a healthcare provider, can help optimize results.

Summary

Oral peptides represent a promising and increasingly accessible approach to improving health, supporting recovery, regulating hormones, and sharpening cognitive function—all without the invasiveness of injections. These formulations offer the convenience of capsules, tablets, or sublinguals, making them appealing for individuals seeking the benefits of peptide therapy without medical supervision or complex delivery systems.

While the bioavailability of oral peptides can vary depending on formulation and digestive factors, advancements in encapsulation and delivery technologies are significantly enhancing their effectiveness.

When taken consistently and with the proper dosage, oral peptides can support a wide range of goals, from boosting growth hormone levels and enhancing fat metabolism to improving skin elasticity, joint function, and even mood stability. Additionally, the strategic stacking of different peptides—combining complementary compounds—can amplify results, especially when tailored to an individual's health status, age, and lifestyle.

That said, results are not immediate or guaranteed. Patience and monitoring are essential, as the body may respond subtly over time. Those who experience the most benefit typically pair peptide use with other foundational health strategies, such as proper nutrition, regular exercise, and adequate sleep.

In the next section, we will turn our focus to injectable peptides—examining how they compare to oral formulations in terms of absorption, precision, and therapeutic power. We'll discuss why some peptides work better when injected, what conditions may warrant a more direct approach, and how to safely integrate injectables into a comprehensive peptide protocol for accelerated healing, performance enhancement, and long-term vitality.

Segment 3: Injectable Peptides (Expanded Guide)

Injectable peptides are among the most effective delivery methods available in the realm of regenerative medicine and advanced wellness. Unlike oral peptides, which must survive digestion and be absorbed through the gut, injectables offer a direct pathway into the bloodstream. This results in greater bioavailability and faster results—critical for those seeking rapid healing, optimized hormone levels, and robust metabolic changes.

Understanding Injectable Peptides

Injectable peptides are administered either subcutaneously (just under the skin) or intramuscularly (into muscle tissue). This method bypasses the digestive system, allowing the peptide to retain its structure and function. These peptides work by mimicking naturally occurring sequences that signal the body to initiate repair, stimulate hormone production, reduce inflammation, and more.

Because of their precision and potency, injectable peptides are widely used in clinical settings for conditions like soft tissue injuries, chronic fatigue, hormone deficiencies, and metabolic resistance. At Delgado Labs, we emphasize safety, education, and results—ensuring users are empowered to use injectables with confidence.

Key Benefits of Injectables:

- **Maximum absorption:** Near-complete uptake compared to oral peptides
- **Faster onset of action:** Especially valuable post-surgery or during flare-ups
- **Tissue-targeting potential:** Injections near injury sites can accelerate healing
- **Hormonal balance:** Especially useful for stimulating endogenous growth hormone and improving testosterone/estrogen ratios indirectly

Injectable peptides offer nearly complete absorption compared to pills, faster healing after surgery or injury, the ability to target specific tissues, and natural hormone balancing (growth hormone, testosterone, estrogen).

BPC-157: Helps heal tendons, joints, gut lining, and reduces inflammation; promotes blood vessel growth and speeds up cellular repair; dose is about 5–10 tiny syringe marks

(0.05–0.1 mL) once or twice daily into belly fat or near injury; best stacked with TB-500 for faster recovery; cycle 4–6 weeks on, 1–2 weeks off.

TB-500: Supports muscle repair, improves joint flexibility, and reduces scar tissue; stimulates actin for better healing; dose is 20–40 syringe marks (0.2–0.4 mL) split across 2–3 shots per week (e.g., Mon/Wed/Fri); cycle 4–6 weeks on, 2 weeks off.

CJC-1295 + Ipamorelin: Boosts growth hormone naturally for anti-aging, better sleep, fat burning, and muscle protection; dose is 5–10 syringe marks (0.05–0.1 mL) each before bed or after workouts; use for 12–16 weeks, then take 4 weeks off; avoid if cancer or uncontrolled diabetes is present.

Sermorelin: Stimulates your body's own growth hormone release, ideal for age-related decline; dose is 5–10 syringe marks (0.05–0.1 mL) nightly; cycle for 3–6 months.

AOD-9604: Speeds fat loss without altering natural growth hormone; inject 10 syringe marks (0.1 mL) daily into belly fat; cycle 8–12 weeks, then rest.

Semaglutide: Controls hunger, insulin, and supports weight loss; mimics GLP-1 hormone to slow digestion; start with 5 syringe marks (0.05 mL) once weekly and increase slowly; use long-term under supervision to avoid nausea.

*__Tip__: Combine with DHA or Alpha-GPC for amplified brain benefits

- Injectable Peptides can work within days. For this and many other reasons we advocate doing microdosing when using injectable Peptides.
- The easiest way to do **microdosing** is to fill up the vial of peptide powder to the top of the vial with bacteriostatic water. Then use little as possible starting in sensitive individuals with less than .10 units which is 5 units on the insulin syringe needle.

- Then after 2 weeks gradually increase the amount to 10 units and not much above 20 units. When using too high a dose many report feeling nausea which goes away.

Smart Stacking: Recovery Stack (BPC-157 + TB-500); Fat-Burning Stack (AOD-9604 + Semaglutide); Growth Stack (CJC-1295 + Ipamorelin + Sermorelin); monitor for overlapping effects.

Cycling and Safety: Cycle short-term repair peptides 4–6 weeks, growth hormone peptides 12–16 weeks; rotate injection sites (left/right belly, thigh, glute) to avoid irritation;

monitor with labs like IGF-1, cortisol, fasting glucose, thyroid.

Note those with extremely low cortisol levels at various times in the morning or afternoon proceed cautiously, when using growth hormone releasing peptides.

Those with symptoms of chronic fatigue are approaching Addison's disease or inability to produce sufficient cortisol, an important catabolic hormone that must remain in balance with Highly anabolic peptides, Testosterone and thyroid can create further aggravation enough that a person could feel faint, vomit, and take days to recover from.

This is another reason that it's best when using injectable peptides to be under a doctor's care. If you have any of these symptoms it is best to do your research and be tested for adrenal fatigue.

Real-World Results: BPC-157 + TB-500 helped a 54-year-old athlete recover from rotator cuff surgery in 5 weeks; CJC-1295 + Ipamorelin boosted a 42-year-old executive's energy, sleep, and focus within 3 weeks; Semaglutide + AOD-9604 helped a 63-year-old lose 14 lbs in 2 months and improve blood markers.

Monitoring: Track energy, body composition, and recovery using journals or fitness trackers; adjust dosage if needed; watch for side effects like water retention (MK-677), nausea (Semaglutide), or sleep issues (high GH peptides).

Note: semiglutide is marketed as Ozempic which is a long acting GLP one agonist to treat type two diabetes.

The use of Wegovy orally has been used successfully with long-term weight management.

Retatrutide (Ray-Tat Tra-tide) is nicknamed **GLP-3** targets **three** receptors GLP-1, GIP and Glucagon.

https://www.instagram.com/reel/DR-kPM8khZp/?igsh=MzRlODBiNWFlZA==

It is considered the next generation in weight loss because in trials by Eli Lilly (not yet FDA approved) the weight reduction is higher (up to 24 to 29% in studies) compared to GLP-1 which only targets one receptor site, and GLP-2 which targets 2 receptors sites. Dr William Seeds MD told Dr Nick Delgado that the Glucagon in GLP3 Retatrutide is exciting to help when used in microdosing and a sensible diet and exercise plan to target more fat reduction while building lean muscle mass.

Summary:

Cycling and Safety

Cycling helps prevent receptor desensitization and maintains long-term efficacy. Example cycling principles:

- Short-Term Repair (4–6 weeks): BPC-157, TB-500
- Hormonal Support (12–16 weeks): CJC-1295, Sermorelin
- Chronic Use with Medical Supervision: Semaglutide

Injection rotation is key to preventing site irritation. Alternate between left and right sides of the abdomen, thigh, or glute.

Real-World Applications and Results

At Delgado Protocol, we've supported doctors treating thousands of clients with personalized peptide regimens. Here are a few case examples:

Case 1: Torn Rotator Cuff A 54-year-old male athlete used BPC-157 and TB-500 post-surgery. Within 5 weeks, pain had significantly reduced, and mobility was restored beyond expectations. Physical therapy was enhanced due to accelerated collagen repair.

Case 2: Fatigue and Brain Fog A 42-year-old female executive began CJC-1295 + Ipamorelin after reporting poor sleep and hormonal imbalance. By week 3, she reported improved mood, increased energy, and better mental clarity.

Case 3: Metabolic Reset A 63-year-old with insulin resistance used Semaglutide and AOD-9604 under supervision. Lost 14 lbs in 2 months, saw improved blood sugar levels, and reduced triglycerides. Follow-up labs confirmed improvements in metabolic markers.

Monitoring and Optimization

- **Track metrics:** Use fitness trackers or journals for body composition, energy levels, and recovery times
- **Adjust dosage:** Based on lab markers or subjective results
- **Watch for side effects:** Water retention (MK-677), nausea (Semaglutide), or sleep disturbances (high GH peptides)

Work with a practitioner familiar with peptides to monitor IGF-1, cortisol, fasting glucose, and thyroid levels where applicable.

Summary

Injectable peptides deliver unmatched potency and precision for those ready to take their health optimization seriously. While they require more commitment than oral peptides, their clinical results speak volumes. From fat loss and muscle growth to faster healing and enhanced sleep, injectables are a foundational tool in regenerative health. Use wisely, cycle responsibly, and always build on a base of great lifestyle habits.

Segment 4: Additional Peptides (Educational Purposes Only)

While Delgado Protocol focuses on peptides with a well-documented safety and clinical usage profile, it is important to be aware of additional research peptides that are generating interest across the scientific and wellness communities. These compounds, though not currently part of our direct offering, have shown promise in various experimental and early clinical studies. This chapter explores their potential applications, mechanisms, and theoretical protocols.

The Rise of Research-Based Peptides

Peptides such as Selank, Semax, Thymosin Alpha-1, and GHK-Cu represent a new frontier in neuromodulation, immune enhancement, and cosmetic regeneration. Many of these compounds are under investigation in countries like Russia, Israel, and parts of Europe. Their unique mechanisms complement the more common growth hormone secretagogues and tissue repair peptides seen in mainstream functional medicine.

Selank

Selank is a synthetic peptide developed from the naturally occurring tetrapeptide tuftsin. It exhibits anxiolytic (anti-anxiety) effects without sedation, unlike traditional benzodiazepines.

- Primary Uses: Anxiety reduction, immune system modulation
- Mechanism: Influences GABAergic transmission and modulates cytokine activity
- Format: Typically administered nasally
- Clinical Potential: Shown to reduce anxiety while supporting immune balance in clinical settings

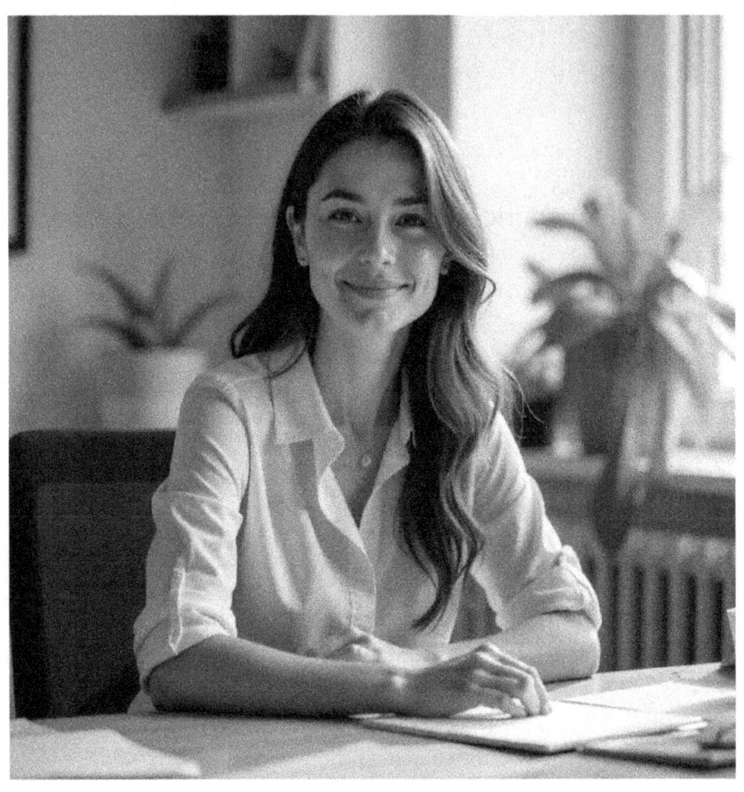

Semax

Semax is a neuropeptide that acts as a cognitive enhancer and neuroprotective agent.

- **Primary Uses:** Cognitive enhancement, brain injury recovery, ADHD
- **Mechanism:** Boosts BDNF (brain-derived neurotrophic factor) and antioxidant enzyme expression
- **Format:** Nasal spray
- **Clinical Note:** Often used after strokes or in neurodegenerative conditions in Russia

DSIP (Delta Sleep-Inducing Peptide)

DSIP promotes natural sleep patterns and may support the regulation of the body's stress and recovery systems.

- **Primary Uses:** Insomnia, sleep disturbances, stress recovery
- **Mechanism:** Believed to influence endogenous opioid peptides and circadian signaling
- **Format:** Injectable or sublingual
- **Observations:** Anecdotal evidence suggests enhanced deep sleep and parasympathetic tone

Thymosin Alpha-1

Thymosin Alpha-1 is a powerful immune peptide used extensively in antiviral protocols.

- **Primary Uses:** Immune restoration, viral infections, chronic fatigue
- **Mechanism:** Enhances T-cell function and interferon production
- **Format:** Injectable (subcutaneous)
- **Clinical Insight:** Studied in cancer and hepatitis C patients for immune resilience

GHK-Cu

GHK-Cu is a copper-binding peptide that supports skin regeneration and may enhance hair and tissue growth.

- **Primary Uses:** Skin rejuvenation, wound healing, anti-aging
- **Mechanism:** Activates tissue remodeling genes, boosts collagen synthesis
- **Format:** Topical cream or injectable
- **Use Case:** Used in cosmetic protocols for wrinkle reduction and scar fading

Tesamorelin

Tesamorelin is a GHRH analog that stimulates natural growth hormone secretion, often used to reduce visceral fat.

- **Primary Uses:** Fat reduction in abdominal area, GH deficiency
- **Mechanism:** Stimulates pituitary to release growth hormone
- **Format:** Injectable
- **FDA Approved For:** HIV-associated lipodystrophy

Experimental Protocol Considerations

While promising, these peptides should only be used under supervision when possible. Recommended guidelines are based on observational and clinical study reviews. Users should:

- Start with minimum effective dose
- Use 5-on 2 days off weekly schedules or 4-week cycles
- Track cognitive, metabolic, immune, or dermatologic changes
- Stacking examples:
- **Neuro Stack:** Semax + Dihexa
- **Immunity Stack:** Thymosin Alpha-1 + Selank
- **Skin Repair Stack:** GHK-Cu + BPC-157 (injectable or topical)

Emerging Peptides and Future Directions

Peptide research is evolving rapidly. Innovations like PEGylation and nanoparticle delivery may soon allow even fragile peptides to be used orally or transdermally. Researchers are exploring peptides that mimic insulin, reduce chronic inflammation, and even extend telomeres for longevity.

As the field matures, we anticipate these compounds will either join mainstream practice or influence the next generation of bioactive therapeutics. For now, education, caution, and professional oversight remain the most important tools when working with novel peptides.

Segment 5: Expert Insights from the Delgado Video Channel

Peptides are more than biochemical compounds—they're real-life tools that have transformed the lives of thousands, including high-performance athletes, aging adults, and patients battling chronic conditions. In this chapter, we synthesize the most important lessons learned from live interviews, conversations, and clinical observations with thought leaders in the peptide field.

These insights were gathered through years of collaboration between Dr. Nick Delgado and experts like peptide researcher Iman Barr MD, Michael Grossman MD and Joshua Helman MD and neuroscientist like Joseph Maroon MD. The goal? To share practical wisdom that bridges the gap between cutting-edge science and real-world results.

Peptide therapy is most effective when it's personalized. While the science behind each peptide provides a roadmap, expert experience helps you fine-tune the path to optimal health. Both Dr Grossman and Dr Helman emphasize the need to respect the body's hormonal rhythms, stress responses, and recovery timelines. Whether the goal is to restore gut integrity, boost muscle mass, or regenerate neurons, timing and consistency are key.

Iman Bar MD, and Michael Grossman MD are veterans in the peptide space, and shared a groundbreaking view on the use of peptides for recovery. They explained that peptides like **BPC-157 and TB-500** aren't just for elite athletes—they're for anyone recovering from trauma, overtraining, or surgery. Our collective experience shows that stacking these two peptides can dramatically reduce inflammation while accelerating soft tissue repair.

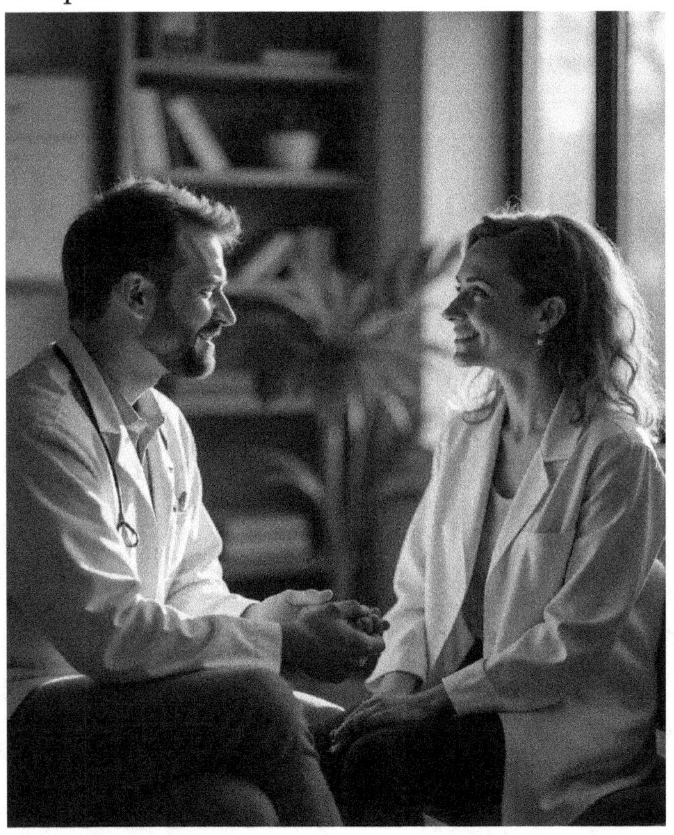

Dr. Nick's Perspective: Real-World Case Reviews

They also emphasized **cycling** peptides to maintain effectiveness. For example, BPC-157 may lose some of its edge if used continually without breaks. A typical schedule: 4 weeks on, 2 weeks off. TB-500, with its systemic action, works best when loaded early and tapered slowly.

Professor Andrew Huberman also addressed the **misuse of peptides**, especially those trying to shortcut the process. After interviewing several experts in the peptide space He warns that poor sourcing and improper dosing can lead to tolerance or even paradoxical effects.

William Seeds MD, founder of SSRP scientific research and performance urges the use of microdosing in his book and my private discussion with his recommendation: start low, stack only when needed, and evaluate outcomes before adding new compounds.

Dr. Nick Delgado contributed his real-life cases to validate Dr Seeds and a bodybuilder named Trevors insights. One example included a competitive weightlifter with chronic elbow tendinitis who used BPC-157 and TB-500 for 8 weeks. The result? Complete resolution of inflammation and a return to training at full intensity without NSAIDs or surgery.

Another case involved a patient recovering from GI surgery. By integrating oral BPC-157 with high-dose probiotics, L-glutamine, and a clean anti-inflammatory diet, the patient not only healed faster but avoided common complications like leaky gut syndrome.

Andrew Huberman & Dr. Nick: Brain Health and Cognitive Peptides

Dr. Huberman, a neuroscientist at Stanford, has extensively studied the brain's response to peptides and neurohormones. In podcasts, Dr. Nick reacted when he highlighted the peptides **Dihexa** and **Semax** as two of the most promising compounds for cognitive enhancement.

Semax, originally developed in Russia, shows promise in boosting **brain-derived neurotrophic factor (BDNF)**—a protein that helps grow and repair neurons. Dihexa, on the other hand, stimulates synaptic plasticity and may be helpful in recovering memory after traumatic brain injury or cognitive decline.

The key insight from Huberman: **brain peptides work best when supported by behavioral habits**. This includes:

- Morning sunlight exposure
- Regular aerobic exercise
- Omega-3 and choline-rich diets
- Proper sleep (with peptides like DSIP or Epitalon as support)

He also warns about overstimulation—some cognitive peptides may cause **mental fatigue or irritability** when used daily. His advice: use brain peptides in cycles, allow neural rest days, and use sleep-enhancing peptides to balance excitation.

Guiding Principles from the Experts

From the collective wisdom of William Seeds, Edwin Lee MD Endocrinologist, Huberman, and Delgado, we derive five key principles:

1. Start Low, Go Slow - Especially for cognitive peptides and GH secretagogues.
2. Cycle Wisely - Avoid burnout or loss of efficacy with strategic on/off patterns.
3. Use Quality Sources - Avoid gray market peptides that may be contaminated or underdosed.

4. Stack with Purpose - Don't stack for the sake of complexity. Combine peptides with synergy and intention.
5. Support the Protocol - No peptide can override poor sleep, diet, or lifestyle habits.

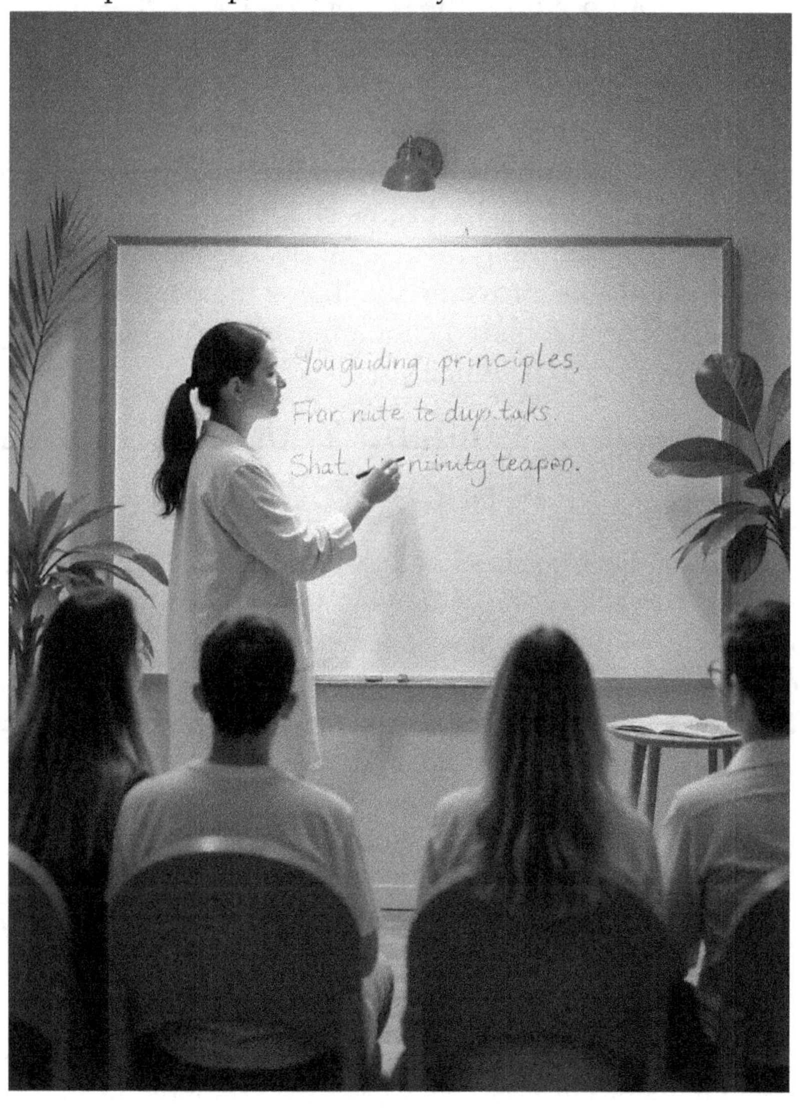

Final Word: Peptides and Personalized Medicine

Peptides are ushering in a new era of **personalized, regenerative health care**. As Dr Lee said in his interview, "Peptides aren't magic. They're tools. But the more precise your tool, the more beautiful the sculpture." Dr. Nick echoed this, reminding listeners that peptides work best when paired with a mindset of **progress over perfection**.

Whether you're recovering from injury, pursuing longevity, or optimizing brain performance, the guidance in this book—and especially in this chapter—can help you take your first or next step with confidence. Always consult a trusted healthcare provider familiar with peptide protocols, and remember: the body is not a machine to be hacked. It's a dynamic system to be tuned.

Segment 6: Building Your Personalized Peptide Protocol

Designing a personalized peptide protocol is a strategic process that allows individuals to take control of their health by using peptides to achieve specific goals such as recovery, fat loss, muscle growth, cognitive enhancement, and longevity. Peptides, which are short chains of amino acids that function as signaling molecules in the body, provide a natural, targeted way to address health concerns by mimicking the body's own processes. By tailoring a protocol to your unique needs and lifestyle, you can maximize the benefits of peptide therapy and optimize your health in a way that fits your individual goals.

1. Defining Your Health Goals

Before you can begin selecting peptides, it's crucial to define your primary health goals. Are you looking to recover faster from an injury? Boost your metabolism and lose fat? Improve your cognitive function? Or are you focused on slowing the aging process and enhancing longevity? Each goal will require a slightly different approach, and understanding your objective is the first step in designing an effective peptide protocol.

For instance:

- Recovery: If recovery is your goal, you might focus on peptides that enhance tissue repair, reduce inflammation, and support cellular regeneration, such as BPC-157, TB-500, and GHRP-2.
- Fat Loss: To support fat loss, peptides like AOD-9604, Semaglutide, and MK-677 may be ideal choices, as they help regulate metabolism, improve fat burning, and stimulate growth hormone production.
- Muscle Growth and Performance: For muscle building and improving athletic performance, CJC-1295, Ipamorelin, MK-677, and PEG-MGF can be used to stimulate growth hormone release, enhance muscle recovery, and improve endurance.
- Cognitive Enhancement: If enhancing brain function and cognitive clarity is your primary focus, peptides like Dihexa, Semax, and Noopept can support neuroplasticity, memory retention, and cognitive clarity.
- Longevity and Anti-Aging: For longevity and anti-aging, Epitalon, Thymosin Beta-4, and NAD+ precursors like NMN or NR are frequently utilized to support DNA repair, cell regeneration, and energy production at the cellular level.

By identifying your specific health goals, you will be able to choose peptides that align with your desired outcomes.

2. Selecting the Right Peptides for Your Protocol

Once you have defined your health goals, the next step is to choose the peptides that will help you achieve those goals.

Peptides can be broadly categorized based on their effects on different systems in the body—such as growth hormone release, tissue repair, fat loss, cognitive function, and longevity. Understanding the mechanisms of action behind each peptide is essential in making the right choice for your personalized protocol.

2 Peptides for Recovery and Healing:

- BPC-157: Known for its powerful healing effects, BPC-157 is often used to accelerate tissue repair, reduce inflammation, and heal soft tissues like ligaments, tendons, and muscles. It has been shown to promote angiogenesis (new blood vessel growth), which is crucial for healing.
- TB-500 (Thymosin Beta-4): This peptide also plays a role in tissue repair, particularly for muscle recovery. It is commonly used to reduce inflammation, promote collagen synthesis, and enhance cell migration for faster recovery from injuries.
- GHRP-2 (Growth Hormone Releasing Peptide-2): This peptide stimulates the pituitary gland to release growth hormone, which can aid in muscle repair, fat burning, and overall recovery.

3 Peptides for Fat Loss and Metabolism:

- AOD-9604: A fragment of human growth hormone, AOD-9604 specifically targets fat cells by stimulating lipolysis (fat breakdown) without affecting growth hormone levels. It is ideal for targeted fat loss, particularly around stubborn fat areas.
- Semaglutide: A GLP-1 agonist, Semaglutide helps regulate appetite and insulin sensitivity, promoting weight loss by reducing hunger and improving

metabolism. It is particularly effective for individuals who struggle with metabolic resistance.

- MK-677 (Ibutamoren): MK-677 is a potent secretagogue that stimulates growth hormone release, promoting muscle growth, fat loss, and improved sleep. It can be particularly beneficial for people looking to optimize muscle mass while reducing body fat.

4 Peptides for Muscle Growth and Performance:

- CJC-1295: A growth hormone-releasing hormone (GHRH) analog, CJC-1295 increases the secretion of growth hormone in the body, leading to enhanced muscle growth, fat loss, and improved recovery. It is often stacked with Ipamorelin for synergistic effects.
- Ipamorelin: This peptide stimulates the pituitary gland to produce more growth hormone, leading to improved muscle mass, recovery, and fat loss. It is often combined with CJC-1295 to achieve a more sustained release of growth hormone.
- PEG-MGF (Mechano Growth Factor): This peptide promotes muscle growth by stimulating the production of proteins that support muscle regeneration. It is especially useful for individuals recovering from muscle injuries or those looking to maximize hypertrophy.

5 Peptides for Cognitive Enhancement:

- Dihexa: Dihexa is a potent cognitive enhancer that promotes neuroplasticity and synaptic growth. It can help improve memory, learning, and overall brain function, making it ideal for those looking to enhance mental clarity and cognitive performance.
- Semax: This peptide has neuroprotective properties and can help enhance cognitive function by increasing levels

of brain-derived neurotrophic factor (BDNF). It is particularly beneficial for individuals with age-related cognitive decline or those seeking mental clarity and focus.

- Noopept: Similar to Semax, Noopept improves cognitive function by increasing BDNF and enhancing synaptic plasticity. It is often used to boost memory, learning capacity, and focus.

6 Peptides for Longevity and Anti-Aging:

- Epitalon: Epitalon is a peptide that stimulates the production of telomerase, the enzyme responsible for the repair and lengthening of telomeres. Telomeres shorten as we age, and their preservation can help extend lifespan and slow the aging process. Epitalon is commonly used in anti-aging protocols to promote cellular regeneration.
- NAD+ Precursors (NMN, NR): Nicotinamide Mononucleotide (NMN) and Nicotinamide Riboside (NR) are precursors to NAD+ (Nicotinamide Adenine Dinucleotide), a coenzyme that plays a critical role in energy production and DNA repair. As we age, NAD+ levels decrease, which can accelerate the aging process. Supplementing with NAD+ precursors can support energy production, enhance cellular repair, and improve overall longevity.

7 Bicycling Peptides for Maximum Effectiveness

Cycling peptides is an essential part of any personalized protocol. Just as the body requires rest periods between workouts to recover and grow, peptides also require breaks to ensure that they continue to work effectively. Without cycling, the body can become desensitized to the effects of peptides, leading to diminishing returns over time.

The most common cycling strategies include:

- Short-Term Cycling (4-6 weeks on, 1-2 weeks off): This is ideal for peptides like BPC-157 and TB-500, which are used for recovery and healing. After a 4-6 week cycle, taking a short break helps the body reset and maintain the peptides' effectiveness.
- Longer Cycling (12-16 weeks on, 4 weeks off): Peptides like CJC-1295 and Ipamorelin, which promote long-term growth hormone release, benefit from longer cycles. After a 3-4 month period of continuous use, a 4-week break is recommended to prevent receptor desensitization and ensure continued efficacy.
- Seasonal Cycling: Some peptides, particularly those related to aging and recovery, can be cycled seasonally. For example, Epitalon might be used for 20 days on, followed by 10 days off, and then taken again after a few months for its anti-aging benefits. This strategy allows you to benefit from the peptides' effects while preventing the body from becoming accustomed to them.

Cycling peptides properly ensures that they remain effective and reduces the risk of side effects.

8 Monitoring Progress and Adjusting Your Protocol

Tracking your progress is a key part of a personalized peptide protocol. Regular monitoring allows you to determine if the peptides are achieving the desired effects and whether any adjustments need to be made. There are several ways to track your progress, including physical metrics, subjective feedback, and lab testing.

- Physical Metrics: Track changes in body composition, muscle mass, fat percentage, energy levels, and recovery times. Using tools like body fat calipers, scales, or even

DEXA scans can help you monitor changes in your body's composition.

- Subjective Feedback: Pay attention to how you feel day-to-day. Are you experiencing better sleep? Are your energy levels higher? Are you recovering faster from workouts? Your subjective experience can give valuable insights into how your protocol is working.
- Lab Testing: Periodic lab tests can help you monitor blood markers like IGF-1, growth hormone levels, CRP, and testosterone. These markers provide a more objective measure of how well your protocol is working and whether any adjustments are needed.

Once you have gathered enough feedback, you can adjust the dosage, peptides, or cycling periods as needed. It's important to remember that peptide therapy is dynamic and may require periodic fine-tuning.

9. Integrating Peptides with Lifestyle Habits

Peptides work best when integrated into a holistic wellness plan. Proper nutrition, exercise, and stress management can all enhance the effectiveness of peptide therapy. For example, peptides like MK-677 and CJC-1295 can support muscle growth and recovery, but they work even better when combined with a consistent resistance training program. Similarly, peptides like BPC-157 and TB-500 promote tissue healing, but their effects can be enhanced with proper nutrition and rest.

- Nutrition: A nutrient-dense diet rich in whole foods, healthy fats, lean proteins, and plenty of vegetables can support the body's healing and recovery processes. Supplementing with additional nutrients like collagen, vitamin C, and omega-3 fatty acids can further enhance the effects of peptides like BPC-157 and TB-500.
- Exercise: Regular physical activity, especially resistance training, can amplify the effects of peptides that support

muscle growth and recovery. Peptides like CJC-1295, MK-677, and Ipamorelin are particularly effective when combined with a consistent workout routine.

- Stress Management: Chronic stress can hinder the effectiveness of peptides and slow down recovery. Integrating stress-reducing practices such as meditation, deep breathing, yoga, or mindfulness can improve peptide efficacy and overall health.

I believe firmly guiding my clients with NLP, Neurolinguistic programming, Deep trans phenomena, parts integration, and reworking the "old Story" to a new story using changes in color, size, speed, sound and thoughts which is how all humans store memories according my mentor Richard Bandler PhD and Dr Tad James. This is the basis of part 3 of my coming book to get fantastic lasting results. Part 4 will go into strategy, diet and exercise at the most advanced level.

10. Safety Considerations and Best Practices

While peptides offer significant health benefits, it's essential to follow safety guidelines to ensure their effectiveness and prevent potential side effects. Only use high-quality peptides from reputable sources, and work with a healthcare provider who is knowledgeable about peptide therapy. Avoid using peptides that have not been properly researched or tested, as their safety and efficacy may be unverified.

Also, start with lower doses when beginning a new peptide regimen. This allows your body to acclimate and reduces the risk of adverse reactions. Gradually increase the dosage based on feedback and monitoring.

Lastly, always cycle peptides according to recommended guidelines. Overuse without breaks can lead to receptor desensitization, diminishing the peptides' effectiveness and increasing the likelihood of side effects.

Segment 7: Advanced Peptide Protocols and Case Studies

Introduction

Advanced peptide protocols are designed for individuals who are looking to address specific health challenges or optimize performance at a deeper level. These protocols often involve combining multiple peptides in a strategic manner to target various biological processes simultaneously. By stacking peptides and using them in specific cycles, individuals can achieve more comprehensive and synergistic results. While basic peptide protocols are often sufficient for general health and wellness, advanced protocols allow for more profound, targeted effects, particularly when it comes to recovery from serious injuries, hormone optimization, and performance enhancement.

Understanding Peptide Stacking

Peptide stacking refers to the practice of using multiple peptides together to target different biological pathways, resulting in more comprehensive outcomes. By stacking peptides, individuals can address multiple aspects of their health at once, such as healing, muscle growth, fat loss, and cognitive function. For example, when recovering from a significant injury, combining **BPC-157** and **TB-500** may accelerate both local tissue repair and systemic healing. Similarly, athletes aiming to enhance muscle recovery and growth might use a stack of **CJC-1295** and **Ipamorelin**, which stimulate natural growth hormone release, alongside **MK-677** for sustained growth hormone production. Stacking peptides allows each compound to complement the others, creating a powerful synergy that enhances their individual effects.

The benefits of peptide stacking go beyond merely increasing the quantity of peptides used. When peptides are combined thoughtfully, they can work together in harmony, targeting different biological processes that may otherwise require multiple approaches. This approach ensures that all areas of a health goal are covered, whether that's optimizing recovery, enhancing performance, or supporting cognitive function. By stacking peptides with complementary mechanisms of action, individuals can achieve better, more rapid results.

Peptide Cycling for Advanced Results

Cycling peptides is a practice that helps prevent the body from becoming desensitized to their effects. Just like the body needs rest after exercise to recover and grow, peptides require periods of rest to maintain their effectiveness. Cycling ensures that the body continues to respond to the peptides at optimal levels, without diminishing returns over time. There are several ways to cycle peptides, depending on the specific goals and peptides being used.

For example, a typical peptide cycle might involve using a peptide for 4-6 weeks, followed by a 1-2 week break. This approach prevents receptor desensitization, allowing the body to reset and maintain its response to the peptide. A more extended cycle, such as 90 days of **CJC-1295** and **Ipamorelin**, followed by a 30-day break, may be appropriate for long-term hormone optimization. Cycling also allows individuals to adjust their protocols based on progress and feedback, ensuring they stay on track to achieve their health goals.

Cycling is crucial for maintaining the long-term effectiveness of peptide therapy. It's not just about preventing desensitization; cycling also allows for careful monitoring of progress and adjustments to dosage, timing, and stacks based on how the body is responding. Understanding the principles of cycling can help ensure that peptides continue to deliver results over time and avoid any potential side effects that may arise from constant use.

Case Studies: Real-World Applications

Case studies provide valuable insights into the real-world effectiveness of advanced peptide protocols. These examples showcase how peptides are used to address specific health challenges and demonstrate the tangible benefits that can be achieved with thoughtful protocol design.

Case Study 1: Post-Injury Recovery Protocol A 45-year-old male athlete tore his ACL while training for a marathon. After undergoing surgery, he began a protocol combining **BPC-157** and **TB-500**. Both peptides are known for their ability to accelerate tissue repair and reduce inflammation. Over the course of 6 weeks, the athlete experienced significant pain reduction, increased joint mobility, and faster recovery compared to typical rehabilitation timelines. His physical therapy sessions were more effective due to the enhanced tissue regeneration, and he was able to return to training earlier than expected.

Case Study 2: Hormonal Optimization for Athletes A 30-year-old competitive weightlifter struggled with hormone imbalance and poor muscle recovery, which affected his performance. He began a peptide protocol of **CJC-1295** and **Ipamorelin**, known for their ability to stimulate natural growth hormone production. After following the protocol for 12 weeks, the athlete saw significant improvements in muscle mass, energy levels, and recovery time. His performance in the gym improved, and he reported feeling more energized and focused both during and after workouts.

Case Study 3: Cognitive Enhancement Protocol A 50-year-old executive sought to improve cognitive function and memory, which had been declining over the years due to chronic stress and poor sleep. He adopted a combination of **Dihexa**, **Semax**, and **Epitalon**. Within 3 weeks, he noticed a marked improvement in memory retention, cognitive clarity, and mental sharpness. The peptides supported neurogenesis and synaptic plasticity, which helped his brain function at a higher level, particularly in high-stress work situations. He also reported better sleep quality and a reduction in anxiety.

Case Study 4: Fat Loss and Metabolic Reset A 40-year-old woman who had struggled with weight gain and metabolic resistance turned to **AOD-9604** and **Semaglutide** to help reset her metabolism and improve her insulin sensitivity. Over a period of 8 weeks, she lost 18 pounds, and her blood sugar levels normalized. She also experienced a reduction in visceral fat and an overall improvement in energy levels. This protocol, under medical supervision, helped her regain control over her metabolism and achieve sustainable fat loss.

Case Study 5: General Health and Longevity A 60-year-old man interested in anti-aging and longevity utilized a combination of **CJC-1295**, **Sermorelin**, **Epitalon**, and **NAD+ precursors**. Over a 6-month period, he experienced improvements in energy, sleep quality, and overall vitality. His blood markers showed an increase in **IGF-1** levels, and he felt younger, both physically and mentally. The combination of peptides, along with his commitment to a healthy diet and exercise routine, contributed to his ongoing health and longevity efforts.

Tailoring Advanced Peptide Protocols to Individual Needs

Personalizing peptide therapy is essential for achieving optimal results. Different individuals have different health goals, genetic backgrounds, and metabolic profiles, so their peptide protocols should be tailored accordingly. Age, gender, and specific health conditions all play a role in determining the best peptides to use and how they should be cycled.

For younger individuals, peptides that support muscle growth and recovery, such as **CJC-1295** and **MK-677**, might be more appropriate, while older adults may benefit from peptides like **Epitalon** and **BPC-157**, which support anti-aging and tissue repair. Women may need to use lower doses and cycle more frequently due to hormonal fluctuations, while men may benefit from higher doses or longer cycles for muscle-building and fat-loss goals.

Monitoring progress is key to ensuring that a personalized peptide protocol is effective. Individuals should track metrics such as energy levels, mood, sleep quality, physical performance, and blood markers like **IGF-1** and **CRP**. Feedback from these metrics can help adjust dosages, introduce new peptides, or modify cycling protocols to align with evolving health goals.

Advanced Strategies: Combining Peptides with Other Therapies

Peptide therapy is most effective when combined with other health optimization strategies. Hormone therapy, for instance, can complement peptides by addressing hormonal imbalances that peptides alone may not fully correct. When combining peptides with bioidentical hormone replacement therapy (HRT), for example, individuals can achieve more comprehensive hormone balance and optimize overall health.

Exercise, particularly strength training, can enhance the effects of peptides like **CJC-1295**, **MK-677**, and **BPC-157**, which support muscle growth and recovery. Pairing peptide therapy with resistance training can accelerate muscle development, fat loss, and recovery times. Additionally, integrating peptides with proper nutrition, especially a high-protein, nutrient-dense diet, can maximize their effectiveness by supporting tissue repair, fat loss, and overall health.

Potential Risks and Considerations

Peptides, though powerful and promising in their therapeutic applications, are not without risks. As biologically active compounds, their benefits depend heavily on precise dosing, quality control, and appropriate medical supervision. The most common risk associated with peptide use stems from improper dosing or misuse. Without proper guidance, users may experience side effects such as water retention, fatigue, or hormonal imbalances. These issues often arise when individuals self-administer peptides in excess doses without understanding their mechanisms of action, half-lives, or interactions with other therapies or medications.

One major concern in the peptide industry is product quality. Peptides sourced from unreliable suppliers may be contaminated, mislabeled, or lack potency. This is especially problematic given that the peptide market remains loosely regulated in many regions. Using substandard peptides can lead to ineffective results or even adverse health outcomes. To mitigate this risk, it's essential to obtain peptides through reputable compounding pharmacies or certified providers and to verify product certificates of analysis (COAs).

We continue to look for the best sources made in USA laboratories third-party tested free of microbes and any contaminants see the reference and updates on ongoing research spanning over 47 years delgadolabs.com.

Long-term use of peptides also requires careful strategy and monitoring. Receptor desensitization can occur if peptides are used continuously without breaks, diminishing their effectiveness over time. To counter this, many clinicians recommend cycling—alternating periods of use with rest periods to allow the body to reset its receptor sensitivity. Regular bloodwork and health assessments should accompany ongoing peptide therapy to detect any emerging side effects or physiological imbalances.

Working with a qualified healthcare provider ensures that peptides are used safely and effectively. A professional can tailor the protocol to an individual's unique needs, monitor progress, and adjust dosages as necessary. When managed responsibly, peptide therapy can deliver exceptional results in anti-aging, cognitive performance, recovery, hormone regulation, and beyond—while minimizing risks and maximizing safety

Segment 8: Advanced Applications and Future Directions of Peptide Therapy

Introduction

Peptide therapy has evolved far beyond its original applications in muscle recovery and injury healing, with advances in biotechnology expanding its potential to address a vast range of health challenges. Over the past decade, peptides have emerged as powerful tools in regenerative medicine, anti-aging therapies, and the treatment of chronic conditions. They are being increasingly used for their ability to target specific cellular functions, enhancing healing processes, reducing inflammation, promoting fat loss, and even supporting cognitive function. With such a wide range of applications, peptides are becoming a cornerstone of personalized and precision medicine, tailored to meet the needs of each individual.

Remember, Peptides are short chains of amino acids (40 Amino Acids) that mimic the body's natural signaling molecules. They work by activating specific receptors in the body, influencing various biological processes that are vital to overall health. Whether it's stimulating the production of growth hormones, repairing damaged tissues, or regulating metabolic functions, peptides offer highly targeted solutions with fewer side effects than traditional medications. As research continues to expand our understanding of peptide biology, new therapies are emerging that promise to change the landscape of healthcare. From treating chronic diseases to improving athletic performance and enhancing longevity, peptides hold the potential to revolutionize modern medicine. This section delves into the advanced applications of peptide therapy, explores the future directions of peptide-based treatments, and highlights the groundbreaking role they are poised to play in the coming decades.

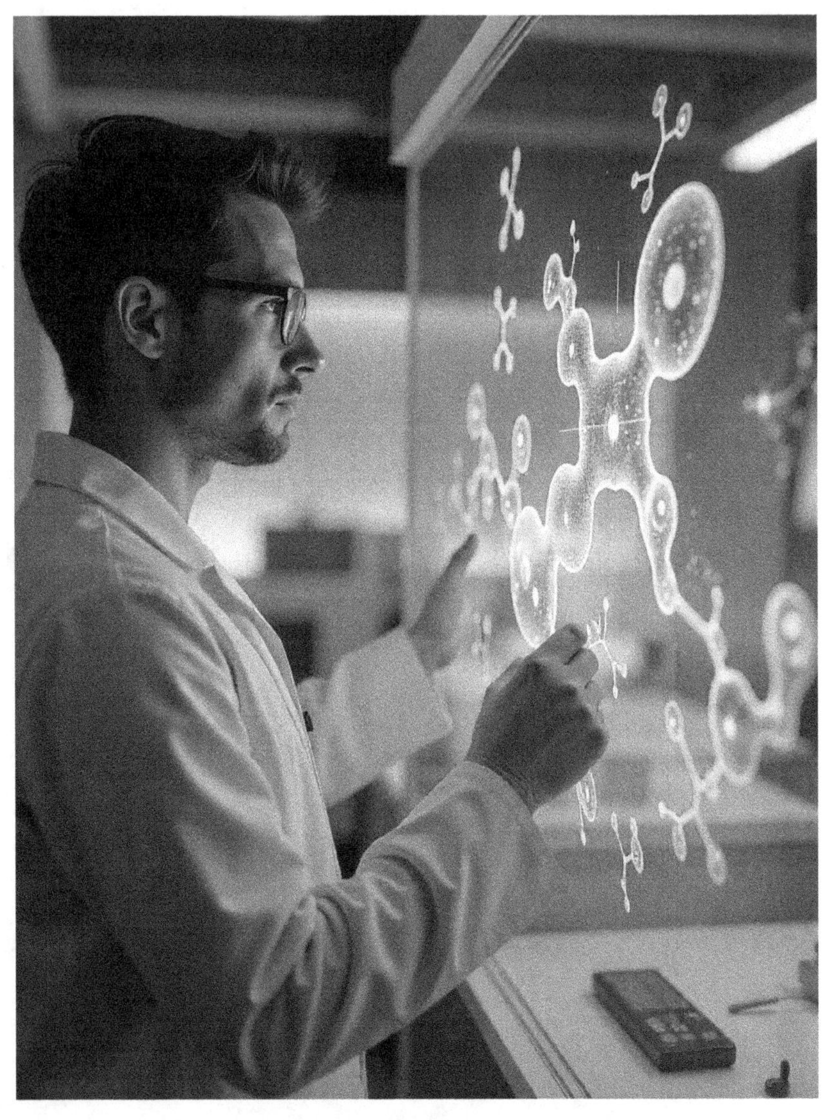

1. Exploring Cutting-Edge Peptide Applications

Peptide Applications in Regenerative Medicine

One of the most exciting applications of peptide therapy is in regenerative medicine, where peptides are used to promote tissue repair, cellular regeneration, and healing. Regenerative medicine seeks to repair or replace damaged tissues and organs, potentially reducing the need for invasive surgeries or long-term treatments. Peptides play a crucial role in this field by accelerating the body's natural healing processes and enhancing recovery from injuries.

Peptides like **BPC-157** (Body Protective Compound-157) and **TB-500** (Thymosin Beta-4) are commonly used in regenerative medicine for their remarkable ability to promote healing. **BPC-157**, in particular, has been studied for its ability to stimulate angiogenesis—the growth of new blood vessels—which is critical for tissue repair. It has been used effectively to accelerate the healing of ligaments, tendons, muscles, and even nerve tissues, reducing recovery times significantly. **TB-500**, another widely used peptide, enhances cell migration and stimulates collagen production, both of which are vital for wound healing and the regeneration of soft tissues. These peptides are also utilized in treating chronic conditions like tendonitis, arthritis, and muscle strains, making them invaluable in the rehabilitation of athletes and individuals recovering from surgeries or injuries.

Another important peptide in regenerative medicine is **Thymosin Beta-4**. It has shown strong potential in promoting the healing of injured tissues, particularly in the cardiovascular system. Research indicates that Thymosin Beta-4 helps regenerate endothelial cells, which are essential for the formation of new blood vessels. This makes it a key player in healing wounds, particularly in patients with chronic ulcers or severe cardiovascular damage.

Peptides are also being explored in treatments for skin regeneration, with promising results in accelerating wound healing and reducing scar formation. The ability to stimulate growth and rejuvenation of tissues has profound implications for both acute injury and the chronic conditions that come with aging, such as joint degradation and tendon weakening.

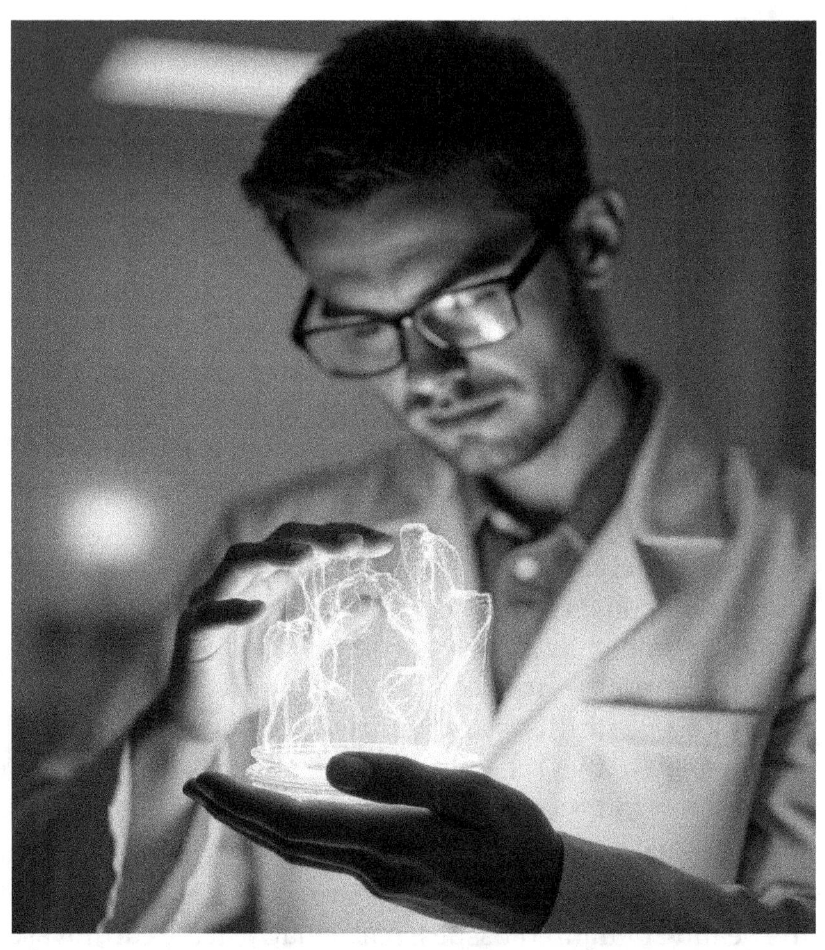

Peptide-Based Therapies for Chronic Conditions

Peptides are making their way into therapies for chronic diseases that have been difficult to treat with conventional medications. **AOD-9604**, a peptide fragment derived from human growth hormone, is one such example. Initially developed for obesity treatment, **AOD-9604** has shown promising results in improving fat metabolism by stimulating the breakdown of fat cells without affecting blood glucose levels. This peptide offers a safer alternative to traditional fat-burning medications, making it an attractive option for those struggling with metabolic conditions like obesity and type 2 diabetes.

For diabetes, peptides like **Semaglutide**, a **GLP-1** receptor agonist, are now being used as part of a revolutionary approach to regulate insulin sensitivity and improve blood sugar levels. Semaglutide helps to reduce appetite, slow gastric emptying, and enhance insulin secretion in response to food intake, making it effective in the treatment of both diabetes and obesity. Clinical trials have demonstrated significant improvements in weight loss and blood glucose regulation, making it a breakthrough in managing metabolic disorders.

Additionally, peptides are showing promise in treating autoimmune diseases. **Thymosin Alpha-1** is a peptide that modulates the immune system and has been used to treat autoimmune disorders by boosting the body's natural defense mechanisms. It works by stimulating the production of T-cells, which are critical for immune responses and pathogen defense. Clinical trials have shown that **Thymosin Alpha-1** can help reduce the severity of autoimmune diseases like chronic hepatitis and even improve responses in patients with HIV.

These peptide-based therapies offer a new frontier in treating chronic diseases, offering targeted, precise treatments that minimize side effects compared to traditional medications.

Peptides for Neurodegenerative Diseases

Another groundbreaking application of peptides is in the treatment of neurodegenerative diseases such as Alzheimer's, Parkinson's, and multiple sclerosis. These diseases are characterized by the degeneration of brain cells, leading to cognitive decline and motor dysfunction. Peptides like **Dihexa**, **Semax**, and **Noopept** are at the forefront of research into cognitive enhancement and neuroprotection.

Dihexa, in particular, has gained significant attention for its ability to stimulate synaptic growth and improve neuroplasticity, which refers to the brain's ability to form new neural connections. Studies suggest that **Dihexa** can enhance memory retention, learning, and overall brain function. By promoting the growth of synapses—the connections between neurons—**Dihexa** holds the potential to improve cognitive function in patients suffering from age-related cognitive decline, traumatic brain injuries, or neurodegenerative diseases.

Semax, originally developed in Russia, is a nootropic peptide that has been studied for its neuroprotective and cognitive-enhancing properties. It works by increasing the expression of brain-derived neurotrophic factor (BDNF), a protein that plays a key role in neurogenesis and synaptic plasticity. **Semax** has been shown to improve memory, enhance focus, and protect the brain from oxidative stress, which is particularly beneficial for individuals with Alzheimer's disease or other cognitive disorders.

These peptides offer a novel approach to slowing the progression of neurodegenerative diseases and even reversing some of the cognitive decline associated with aging. While the research is still in its early stages, the results so far have been promising, suggesting that peptides could one day play a central role in maintaining cognitive health and treating conditions like Alzheimer's.

Peptides for Cognitive Function

Cognitive decline is a growing concern as the population ages, and there is increasing interest in peptide therapies that can enhance memory, learning, and overall brain function. Peptides like **Semax**, **Dihexa**, and **Noopept** are already showing promise as cognitive enhancers, and future developments in peptide research may lead to even more potent compounds capable of improving mental performance in both healthy individuals and those with neurodegenerative diseases.

Dihexa, a peptide known for its neurogenic properties, promotes the formation of new synapses in the brain, enhancing neuroplasticity. This peptide has been shown to improve memory and learning capacity, making it a promising candidate for treating conditions like Alzheimer's and other forms of dementia.

Semax, another peptide being explored for its cognitive benefits, has been demonstrated to increase levels of brain-derived neurotrophic factor (BDNF), a protein that plays a crucial role in supporting the growth, survival, and differentiation of neurons. By promoting neurogenesis, Semax has the potential to delay the onset of cognitive decline, improve memory, and reduce the severity of cognitive impairment in aging individuals.

2. Innovative Approaches to Anti-Aging and Longevity

Peptides in Anti-Aging

Peptide therapy has gained immense popularity in the field of anti-aging due to the ability of certain peptides to rejuvenate cells, repair DNA, and reduce the effects of aging. **Epitalon**, a peptide that stimulates telomerase production, is one of the most studied anti-aging peptides. Telomerase is the enzyme responsible for lengthening telomeres, the protective caps at the end of chromosomes. As we age, our telomeres shorten, which leads to cellular senescence (the cessation of cell division) and contributes to the aging process. By activating telomerase, **Epitalon** helps protect telomeres, potentially slowing down or even reversing aspects of cellular aging.

Clinical trials have shown that **Epitalon** can improve the body's overall health, increasing longevity by preventing the degeneration of cellular structures. This peptide has been linked to improvements in sleep quality, immune function, and the regulation of antioxidant enzymes, all of which play a role in maintaining youthfulness.

Peptides like **GHK-Cu** (Copper Peptide) also have significant anti-aging properties, primarily through their ability to stimulate collagen production, reduce wrinkles, and enhance skin regeneration. **GHK-Cu** has been used in various cosmetic formulations for its skin-healing properties, but its systemic effects extend beyond just the skin. It can help improve wound healing, reduce inflammation, and boost the body's ability to repair damaged tissue, making it a powerful tool in maintaining youthful appearance and health.

Peptide Hormone Optimization for Longevity

Growth hormone (GH) is a critical factor in the aging process, as it regulates metabolism, muscle growth, and cellular regeneration. As we age, our natural growth hormone production declines, leading to an increase in body fat, a decrease in muscle mass, and a decline in overall vitality. This is where peptides like CJC-1295 and Ipamorelin come into play. These peptides are growth hormone-releasing hormone (GHRH) analogs, which stimulate the pituitary gland to release more natural growth hormone, thus combating the effects of aging.

CJC-1295, when combined with Ipamorelin, provides a sustained release of growth hormone over an extended period. This not only enhances muscle growth and recovery but also supports fat loss, bone density, and overall vitality. The combination of these peptides can help restore the youthful benefits of growth hormone, making them key players in the fight against aging.

Telomerase Activation: Peptides as Longevity Catalysts

As mentioned, **Epitalon** is a peptide that activates telomerase, helping to preserve the length of telomeres and potentially extending lifespan. This ability to lengthen telomeres is particularly important because telomeres are crucial in determining the lifespan of cells. Shortened telomeres are associated with the aging process and age-related diseases such as cancer, heart disease, and neurodegeneration. By activating telomerase, **Epitalon** provides a way to slow down these processes and improve longevity at the cellular level.

The concept of telomerase activation opens a new frontier in anti-aging medicine. While traditional approaches focused on slowing down the aging process through diet and exercise, peptide therapy presents a more direct method of rejuvenating the body from a cellular perspective. **Epitalon** and similar peptides offer hope for extending lifespan while also improving the quality of life in older individuals.

3. Peptides for Immune System Support

Peptides in Immune Modulation

The immune system plays a vital role in defending the body against infections and diseases, but it can also become dysregulated, leading to autoimmune disorders, chronic inflammation, and reduced immune function. Peptides like **Thymosin Alpha-1** and **Thymosin Beta-4** are now being studied for their ability to modulate the immune system.

Thymosin Alpha-1, in particular, is a peptide that has been shown to enhance the activity of T-cells, which are critical for the immune system's response to infections. It can be used to stimulate the immune system in individuals with compromised immune function or to boost the body's defense mechanisms against chronic infections. **Thymosin Alpha-1** has been shown to be effective in treating conditions like chronic viral infections, HIV, and hepatitis, where traditional treatments may fall short.

Peptides and Chronic Infections

Peptides are also showing promise in the treatment of chronic infections that have been difficult to manage with conventional medications. **Thymosin Alpha-1** has been used in conjunction with other treatments to enhance the immune system's response, helping individuals with chronic infections like hepatitis or even HIV. By boosting the production of T-cells, **Thymosin Alpha-1** helps the body better control and suppress these infections.

This application of peptides offers a potential breakthrough in managing diseases that have long been a challenge for the medical community. As researchers continue to investigate the therapeutic potential of peptides for chronic infections, we may see peptide-based therapies become an integral part of treating viral, bacterial, and fungal infections.

4. Personalized Medicine and Custom Peptide Protocols

How Peptides Are Used in Personalized Medicine

One of the key benefits of peptide therapy is its ability to be customized for each individual. Personalized medicine has become a central focus in modern healthcare, as it allows treatments to be tailored to the unique genetic, environmental, and lifestyle factors of each padividual's tient. Peptides are ideal candidates for personalized treatment because they can be precisely matched to an inspecific health needs.

Using genetic testing and personalized data, healthcare providers can design peptide protocols that are optimized for each patient's unique biology. For example, genetic testing can identify how a person's body responds to growth hormone, which peptides might be most effective for them, and how they should be dosed. This ensures that the peptide therapy is as effective and safe as possible, minimizing risks and maximizing the benefits.

Conclusion

Peptides are rapidly transforming healthcare by offering a new frontier of treatments for chronic conditions, aging, and performance optimization. From regenerative medicine to cognitive enhancement, peptides have demonstrated the ability to target specific biological processes with precision and minimal side effects. The future of peptide therapy is bright, with ongoing research promising even more innovative applications. As we continue to understand the full potential of peptides, they will undoubtedly become a cornerstone of personalized medicine, offering patients the opportunity to take control of their health and achieve optimal well-being. The continued evolution of peptide science will pave the way for groundbreaking therapies that address a wide range of health concerns, from chronic diseases to age-related decline, making peptides one of the most powerful tools in modern medicine.

Segment 9: The Future of Peptide Therapy and Emerging Applications

Introduction

Peptides, once limited to niche applications in the realms of bodybuilding and injury recovery, have experienced rapid expansion in recent years. With new scientific advancements and clinical research, peptides are now recognized for their versatility, targeted action, and potential to revolutionize treatment strategies across multiple areas of medicine. From precision medicine and gene therapy to addressing chronic conditions and enhancing brain health, the future of peptide therapy looks promising, with broad applications still being discovered.

This chapter will explore the future potential of peptide therapy, delving into emerging applications, the role of peptides in precision medicine, novel peptide discoveries, and the integration of cutting-edge technology such as artificial intelligence (AI) and gene editing. We will examine the current challenges and regulatory landscape, as well as the new frontiers that could pave the way for safer, more effective

Personalized Peptide Therapy

Personalized medicine aims to tailor treatment to the individual characteristics of each patient, rather than adopting a one-size-fits-all approach. In recent years, the integration of peptides into personalized medicine has grown substantially. This integration stems from the peptides' ability to target specific molecular pathways and influence bodily functions with high precision. In the future, we will see peptides being utilized in ways that are customized based on a patient's genetic profile, health history, and environmental factors, ensuring maximum effectiveness while minimizing risks and side effects.

One example of this is the use of **pharmacogenomics**, a field that studies how genes affect a person's response to drugs. Peptides could play a pivotal role in this space by enabling therapies that are specifically designed to match a patient's genetic makeup. By identifying specific genetic markers, clinicians can predict how a patient will respond to a peptide-based treatment and adjust dosages or combinations of peptides accordingly.

Through the use of genetic testing, we can predict whether certain peptide therapies, like **CJC-1295**, **BPC-157**, or **TB-500**, will work more effectively for certain individuals. This could revolutionize chronic disease management, cancer therapy, and hormone optimization, among other medical areas. In the future, clinics might offer advanced peptide therapy protocols that are dynamically adjusted based on continuous biometric data gathered via wearables or lab tests.

Peptides in Age-Related Disease Management

Peptide therapies in the coming years.

1. Peptides and the Evolution of Personalized Medicine

One of the most promising applications of personalized peptide therapy lies in its ability to slow or even reverse the effects of age-related diseases. Age-related diseases, such as Alzheimer's, Parkinson's, osteoporosis, and arthritis, are often linked to the body's inability to regenerate tissue or repair cellular damage efficiently. Peptides such as **Epitalon**, **GHK-Cu**, and **TB-500** are already being explored for their potential to enhance tissue regeneration and prevent the cellular aging process.

Peptides like **Epitalon**, for example, are known to activate **telomerase**, an enzyme that maintains the length of telomeres – the protective caps at the end of chromosomes that shorten as we age. As telomeres shorten, cells become less capable of dividing and repairing, leading to the onset of age-related diseases. By restoring telomere length, **Epitalon** can delay the onset of these conditions and improve quality of life in older individuals.

In the future, personalized peptide therapies could be combined with hormone replacement therapies (HRT) and regenerative medicine to form comprehensive treatment protocols that address the underlying causes of age-related diseases. This approach would enable the slowing down of cellular aging while enhancing tissue regeneration, offering a real opportunity to increase both the lifespan and healthspan of individuals.

2. The Role of Peptides in Gene Therapy

Peptides as Gene Therapy Modulators

Gene therapy has long been considered the next frontier in medicine, with the ability to address the root causes of genetic diseases by correcting defective genes or introducing new ones. Peptides are emerging as a powerful tool in gene therapy, due to their ability to carry genetic material into cells or modulate gene expression. In particular, peptides that act as delivery vehicles for genetic material, known as **gene delivery peptides**, have shown great promise in recent studies.

These peptides work by enhancing the delivery of nucleic acids, such as DNA, RNA, or messenger RNA (mRNA), into cells. The process is vital for efficient gene therapy, as the DNA or RNA must enter the cells where the gene correction or introduction occurs. Peptides like **TAT peptides**, derived from the HIV TAT protein, can cross cell membranes and deliver genetic material to target cells effectively.

In the future, peptides could be used in combination with CRISPR-Cas9 technology to provide highly targeted, efficient, and safe gene editing. This could lead to the correction of genetic mutations that cause diseases such as cystic fibrosis, Duchenne muscular dystrophy, or even genetic forms of cancer. Peptides could facilitate the precise delivery of CRISPR systems, ensuring that the genetic material is delivered to the right cells, potentially reducing the off-target effects that are a concern with current gene-editing techniques.

Moreover, peptide-based gene therapies could also be used to stimulate the expression of therapeutic proteins in the body. For instance, peptides could be used to encourage the production of **insulin**, **growth factors**, or **immune system proteins** to treat conditions like **diabetes**, **osteoporosis**, or **cancer**.

Peptides in Cancer Gene Therapy

One exciting avenue for peptide therapy in the future is its application in cancer treatment. Traditional cancer treatments, such as chemotherapy and radiation, can be harsh on the body and often come with significant side effects. Peptides, however, can be used to deliver cancer-fighting agents directly to tumor cells with remarkable specificity. For example, peptides that target **tumor-associated antigens** could be used to deliver drugs or genetic material to cancer cells, significantly reducing the impact on healthy tissues.

Additionally, certain peptides like **Follistatin**, a naturally occurring peptide that inhibits myostatin (a protein that limits muscle growth), are being studied for their potential to inhibit tumor growth and enhance immune response.

I am unimpressed with its ability to build muscle because the muscle is not tasting strong structure however, this peptide may help in controlling enhancing immune system.

Follistatin's ability to influence the **TGF-β** pathway, which regulates cell proliferation and apoptosis (programmed cell death), makes it a valuable therapeutic target in cancer treatment.

The future of peptide therapy in cancer treatment may involve a combination of peptide delivery systems and targeted therapies, potentially offering a more effective and less toxic treatment alternative to traditional methods.

3. Emerging Peptides for Cognitive Enhancement and Mental Health

Peptides in Mental Health Treatment

Mental health disorders such as depression, anxiety, and post-traumatic stress disorder (PTSD) are increasingly prevalent, and traditional treatments like antidepressants and anti-anxiety medications often come with unwanted side effects. Peptides offer a promising alternative due to their ability to regulate neurotransmitter systems and promote the body's natural healing mechanisms.

For example, **Oxytocin**, known as the "love hormone," is a peptide that plays a role in social bonding, emotional regulation, and stress reduction. It has been shown to improve feelings of well-being, reduce anxiety, and enhance emotional connections in both therapeutic and non-therapeutic settings. Future peptide therapies that target the **oxytocin system** could provide new treatments for individuals suffering from anxiety, depression, and PTSD.

Additionally, peptides like **Selank** and **DSIP** (Delta Sleep-Inducing Peptide) are being researched for their potential to reduce anxiety and improve sleep quality. **Selank**, a synthetic peptide derived from **Tuftsin**, has anxiolytic (anti-anxiety) effects without sedation. By modulating the **GABAergic system**, it reduces anxiety and helps improve mood, making it a viable alternative to benzodiazepines, which have a high potential for abuse and dependence.

4.Technological Integration: AI and Machine Learning in Peptide Therapy

AI-Drie Therapy

The integration of **artificial intelligence (AI)** and **machine learning (ML)** into peptide therapy is opening up new possibilities for optimizing treatment protocols. AI can analyze vast amounts of health data, including genetic information, lab results, and patient-reported symptoms, to create highly personalized peptide regimens that are tailored to the unique needs of each patient.

AI systems could also continuously monitor the patient's progress and adjust the peptide therapy in real-time. For instance, by analyzing biomarkers such as **IGF-1 levels**, **growth hormone secretion**, and other relevant metrics, AI could make real-time recommendations about when to change peptide doses, switch peptide types, or cycle between different peptides.

In addition, AI can be used to predict the effectiveness of certain peptides for specific conditions based on a patient's genetic profile. By analyzing historical data from clinical trials and real-world patient data, AI can identify which peptides will likely provide the best outcomes, minimizing trial and error in peptide therapy.

The Role of AI and Technology in Peptide Therapy

The use of artificial intelligence (AI) in peptide therapy is revolutionizing personalized medicine. AI-driven platforms can analyze vast amounts of health data, including genetic information, lab results, and lifestyle factors, to create optimized peptide protocols for individual patients. These systems can suggest the best combinations of peptides, adjust dosages based on real-time data, and track progress over time, offering a level of precision and customization that was previously unattainable.

As technology continues to advance, we can expect AI to play an even more significant role in peptide therapy, allowing for truly personalized, dynamic treatment regimens that evolve with the patient's needs.

Wearables and Continuous Data Collection

Another area where technology will play a significant role is in the development of wearable devices that continuously collect health data. These devices can track parameters such as heart rate variability (HRV), sleep patterns, physical activity, and even blood glucose levels, all of which can inform decisions regarding peptide therapy. Combining wearables with AI-driven analysis could create a real-time feedback loop, allowing clinicians to make data-driven adjustments to peptide treatments on a personalized basis.

The future of peptide therapy could involve patients wearing smart devices that collect and transmit data about their physical and mental health. This would allow healthcare providers to fine-tune treatments, ensuring the peptides are working optimally without the need for frequent in-person visits.

5. Peptides and Global Health

Peptide Therapy in Low-Resource Settings

Peptide therapies, while typically considered cutting-edge, could have significant applications in low-resource settings as well. Many diseases prevalent in low-income and developing countries, such as tuberculosis, malaria, and HIV, are chronic and require long-term management. Peptides like **Thymosin Alpha-1** and **BPC-157** could be used in these regions to support immune function, accelerate wound healing, and improve overall health outcomes.

Additionally, peptide-based treatments may provide cost-effective alternatives to traditional treatments for diseases such as **HIV/AIDS** and **malaria**, where access to conventional medicine is limited. In countries with underdeveloped healthcare systems, peptide therapy could be used to bridge the gap, offering treatments that are effective and accessible.

Conclusion

The future of peptide therapy is both exciting and expansive. As we move forward, peptides will continue to play a critical role in medicine, offering highly targeted, personalized treatments for a wide array of conditions. From gene therapy and chronic disease management to cognitive enhancement and anti-aging, the potential for peptides to transform healthcare is immense. With continued research, technological advancements, and regulatory improvements, peptide therapy is set to become an integral part of modern medicine, providing patients with more precise, effective, and personalized treatment options than ever before.

Segment 10: The Future of Peptide Therapy — Unlocking Human Potential

Peptides are now being used to support fat loss, improve muscle growth, enhance libido, reduce inflammation, reverse signs of aging, and even regenerate damaged tissues. Therapies once limited to elite athletes or anti-aging clinics are becoming accessible to a wider population.

Looking ahead, the future of peptide science holds the potential for profound impact: regenerative healing without surgery,real-time optimization of human performance. As biotech tools continue to improve, peptides may soon become central not just to medical treatment, but to everyday wellness—a new frontier in enhancing human potential.

The Evolution of Peptides: Healing to Enhancement

. Over time, as new peptides were discovered and synthesized, their uses expanded. Clinicians began to appreciate their roles in weight loss, cognitive enhancement, immune resilience, skin repair, sexual health, and metabolic optimization..

Smart Peptides

The Synergy of Peptides, Gene Editing, Exosomes, and Stem Cells

Future health optimization will not rely on a single therapy – it will be synergistic. Peptides will increasingly be used alongside gene editing tools like CRISPR, regenerative therapies involving exosomes, and stem cell infusions.

Exosomes, tiny vesicles secreted by cells, carry signaling molecules that orchestrate regeneration. When combined with regenerative peptides like BPC-157 or thymosin beta-4, exosomes can deliver a double punch: initiating repair and providing the necessary biochemical instructions to sustain it.

Similarly, peptides could be used to "precondition" stem cells before transplantation, increasing their survival rate, integration, and functional output. By modulating the microenvironment through selective peptides, the engraftment and efficacy of stem cell therapies could skyrocket.

Gene editing, meanwhile, offers the possibility of correcting genetic defects or optimizing certain pathways permanently. Peptides could support the gene editing process, either by enhancing DNA repair mechanisms pos t-editing or by modulating immune responses to prevent rejection or unintended consequences.

Together, these technologies represent a layered strategy for rejuvenation and enhancement, far beyond what any single intervention could accomplish.

Personalized Peptide Protocols: Medicine Tailored to You

In the future, peptide therapy will become radically personalized.

Imagine wearable devices that constantly monitor biomarkers like cortisol, inflammation markers. This real-time data could feed into an AI platform that adjusts your peptide dosages and schedules automatically.

Your "peptide protocol" might change from week to week.

- Following a minor injury at the gym, the system might deploy regenerative peptides to accelerate healing.
- In periods of high mental strain, cognitive-enhancing peptides might be prioritized.

This dynamic, living form of therapy would make static prescriptions – take X mg daily for 12 weeks – seem primitive by comparison.

Peptides and the Anti-Aging Dream

For decades, scientists have sought the holy grail: a way to slow, halt, or even reverse aging. While many compounds have been proposed – resveratrol, metformin, rapamycin – none has the versatility and tissue-targeting specificity of peptides.

Anti-aging peptides can work on multiple levels:

- **Mitochondrial health**: Peptides like SS-31 optimize mitochondrial function, reducing oxidative damage.
- **Hormonal balance**: Peptides such as CJC-1295 + Ipamorelin stimulate endogenous growth hormone production without disrupting natural rhythms.
- **Immune modulation**: Thymic peptides enhance immune surveillance, reducing vulnerability to infections and cancer.
- **Tissue regeneration**: BPC-157 and TB-500 accelerate repair of joints, tendons, muscles, and internal organs.
- **Cognitive preservation**: Cerebrolysin-like peptides support neuronal survival, plasticity, and cognitive resilience.

Future protocols could combine dozens of peptides into synergistic regimens designed not just to maintain youthfulness but to gradually rejuvenate aged tissues.

In clinical trials, early evidence suggests that carefully layered peptide therapies can improve telomere length, enhance DNA repair, increase autophagy (cellular cleanup), and restore youthful gene expression profiles. These changes hint at the possibility of true biological age reversal.

Ethical Considerations in the Peptide Era

As peptides move from therapy to enhancement, ethical questions become inevitable:

- Should enhancement be available to all, or only those who can afford it?
- Where is the line between medicine and performance enhancement?
- How do we prevent misuse or over-reliance on biotechnological shortcuts?
- What safeguards are needed to ensure long-term safety in self-experimenters and biohackers?

Medical authorities, governments, and society at large will need to grapple with these questions. While the democratization of peptide access could empower billions to live longer, healthier lives, it could also exacerbate existing inequalities if access is limited by wealth or geography.

Moreover, as amateur biohackers increasingly experiment with peptides bought online, the risk of poorly designed protocols, contamination, and adverse effects grows. Clear guidelines, education, and oversight will be critical to avoid setbacks that could tarnish the reputation of an otherwise life-transforming technology.

Peptides and the Redefinition of Human Limits

In the coming decades, peptides could redefine what it means to be human.

We may see athletes who recover from injuries in days instead of months. Elderly individuals may remain mentally sharp and physically capable well into their 90s or 100s. Chronic diseases that once ravaged bodies could be managed or reversed with multi-layered peptide regimens.

But perhaps most profoundly, peptides could allow individuals to continuously evolve — adapting to new challenges, stresses, and environments with internal flexibility previously reserved for the young and the exceptionally healthy.

Rather than peaking in their 20s or 30s and declining thereafter, humans of the future may experience multiple peaks throughout life, each one ushered in by intelligently designed regenerative therapies.

Preparing for the Peptide Revolution

Whether you are a healthcare provider, a patient, or a wellness enthusiast, the time to prepare for the peptide revolution is now.

- **Stay educated**: Peptide science is evolving rapidly. New discoveries, safety data, and best practices emerge every year.
- **Work with qualified professionals**: Self-experimentation can be valuable but dangerous without proper guidance. Partnering with experienced practitioners ensures protocols are evidence-based and individualized.
- **Focus on fundamentals**: No peptide can replace a poor diet, chronic stress, or sedentary lifestyle. Peptides are force multipliers, not substitutes.
- **Monitor and adapt**: Regular blood work, biomarker analysis, and clinical assessments are key to optimizing and adjusting peptide therapies.
- **Advocate for access**: As peptides become mainstream, supporting efforts for safe, affordable, widespread access is critical.

Conclusion: A New Era Dawns

Peptides are no longer simply therapeutic agents for a few isolated conditions. They are poised to become the cornerstone of a new era in medicine — an era where health is not the absence of disease but the active pursuit of human flourishing.

In this future, the concept of "normal aging" may fade away, replaced by the expectation of lifelong vitality, resilience, and performance. Peptides, along with other regenerative technologies, will unlock levels of health and human potential that were once confined to mythology and science fiction.

Peptides for Incredible Lovemaking, Longevity, Health, Energy and Happiness

Peptides are an exciting new frontier in medicine. They play a key role in the central nervous system, the brain, hormone regulation, the immune system, tissue healing, DNA repair and more. They have an extremely high safety profile; and their uses and benefits are vast. Read on to discover what they are, what they can do for you, and everything else you need to know in order to start receiving the exceptional benefits of peptides.

Watch these videos for more insight then click the link to get this amazing offer.

Love peptides
https://youtu.be/dPTrXTc2xC8

5 Ways to Energy & Immunity for Life. Peptides, Hormones, Plant Diet Harriet McCoy & Dr Nick (in depth 90 minutes)
https://youtu.be/wRxY8jYJJm0

Peptides for Anti Aging
https://youtu.be/A8X_3PzaMMU

Peptides Regenerate
https://youtu.be/Uihs-8QW43Y

Protein peptides & Testosterone
https://youtu.be/SRAM2wSI5jg

Protein Peptides as We age
https://youtu.be/2iHPbZvpDko

4 Secrets to Peak Performance, world class Olympic bicyclist Harriet McCoy
https://youtu.be/qvVPOGtQEoM

What They Are

Peptides are small proteins that are made up of short chains of amino acids. They control gene expression and they regulate every system in your body. Peptides have different effects on the body depending on which sequence of amino acids they contain. There are several thousand peptides - some fight aging and enhance longevity, others reduce inflammation. Some destroy microbes and fight chronic disease, others boost energy and emotional wellbeing. There are also peptides that can enhance and even restore cognitive health and the immune system; and increase athletic performance and recovery time. And finally, there are peptides that can reverse sexual dysfunction, boost sexual pleasure and performance and take your lovelife to a whole new level.

Key Peptides for Anti Aging, Rejuvenation, Health and Intimacy:

PT141

- Improves libido, pleasure, fantasy, performance and orgasmic intensity.
- Can yield a huge improvement in erectile dysfunction in men.

- Improves sexual performance in men, and can allow them to experience strong, firm erections for up to 45 minutes until one climaxes.
- Men need approximately .20 ml. the first few injections to reduce the feelings of nausea, then work up to .40 ml (that is at the 40-unit line of the syringe needle 50 or 100) if needed for a firmer erection in older men. Be sure to time your loving making activity by taking a small injection about 4 hours before activity and prepare for an incredible experience that feels as if you can make love for hours!
- Helps curtail female sexual dysfunction as the fantasy feeling increases arousal for hours after its use.
- Females only need a very small amount injected, approximately .05 ml.
- Don't take too high of a dose so start slowly as you can always add more later or it will cause temporary nausea.
- Notice it may add to a suntan appearance.

Cerebrolysin

- A combination of peptides.
- Reduces inflammation and neuron cell death.
- Slows down the aging process.
- Is used for brain repair in neurodegenerative diseases.
- Has been found useful in patients with Parkinson's Disease, stroke, traumatic brain injury, Autism, dementia and Alzheimer's.[1]

BPC-157 aids in the prevention of gastric ulcers acts systemically in the digestive tract to combat leaky gut, IBS, gastro-intestinal cramps, and Crohn's disease

help skin burns heal at a faster rate

---

[1] https://www.ncbi.nlm.nih.gov/pmc/articles/PMC4263193/

significantly accelerates reticulin and collagen formation
Promote tendon and ligament healing
Help cure periodontitis

Thymosin-Beta-4

- Boosts your immune system
- Decreases scar tissue formation
- Increases collagen formation
- Calms muscle spasm
- Improved muscle tone
- Increased exchange of substances between cells
- Encourages tissue repair
- Stretches connective tissue
- Helps maintain flexibility
- Reduced inflammation of tissue in joints
- Encourages the growth of new blood cells in tissue
- Increased endurance and strength
- Prevents the formation of adhesions and fibrous bands in muscles, tendons, and ligaments
- Used for hair restoration
- Beneficial in non-alcoholic fatty liver disease

Selank and Semax

- Russian peptides that are bioavailable nasally; which means you can just spray it in the nose.
- Used to improve brain function.[2]

---

[2] https://onlinelibrary.wiley.com/doi/abs/10.1002/%28SICI%291520-6769%28199609%2919%3A2%3C115%3A%3AAID-NRC171%3E3.0.CO%3B2-B

- Helps people with emotional issues such as depression, anxiety, and bipolar disorder.

MIF-1, ACTH, Dihexa

- The research is currently limited but promising - they have been used successfully to help people with depression, bipolar disorder, Alzheimer's disease and PTSD.[3]
- May boost mental stamina, focus, heart health and brain health.[4] [5]

GDF11

- Beneficial in tissue repair.
- Useful in antiaging.
- There are potential health drawbacks; start with minimal dosages, work closely with your doctor and be sensible.

IGF1

- Neuroprotective (protects nerves from damage and degeneration).[6]
- Has nerve regenerative factors and capabilities.
- Helps with muscle regeneration.[7]
- Supports skeletal health.[8]

---

3 https://www.ncbi.nlm.nih.gov/pmc/articles/PMC3829467/
4 https://www.ncbi.nlm.nih.gov/pmc/articles/PMC4201273/
5 https://www.ncbi.nlm.nih.gov/pmc/articles/PMC3829467/
6 https://www.ncbi.nlm.nih.gov/pmc/articles/PMC6367275/
7 https://www.ncbi.nlm.nih.gov/pmc/articles/PMC6367275/
8 https://www.ncbi.nlm.nih.gov/pmc/articles/PMC6367275/

- Helps support cardiovascular health and decrease atherosclerosis risk.[9]

Sermorelin (GHRH) + GHRP 6 and GHRP 2

- Enhanced libido
- A boost physical stamina and energy level
- Increase development of lean body mass through the development of new muscle cells
- Improved sleep quality
- Reduce body fat through lipolysis
- Increase energy and vitality
- Increase strength and endurance
- Accelerates healing from wound or surgery
- Strengthens the heart
- Enhances the immune system
- Increases calcium retention and increases bone density
- Improved immune response
- Improved hair and nail growth
- Improvement in skin elasticity

Growth Hormone and IGF-1

Signs of Deficiency

- Premature aging
- Bowed back
- Reduced height with aging(or since childhood)
- Overweight or obese
- Tired
- Deeply wrinkled forehead

---

[9] https://www.ncbi.nlm.nih.gov/pmc/articles/PMC6367275/

- Thin poorly developed eyebrows
- Droopy upper eyelids
- Thinner nose
- Thin lips
- Tense shoulder muscles
- Droopy muscles
- Men: Gynecomastia
- Men & Women: sagging breasts
- Abdominal obesity
- Droopy belly
- Woman: pregnancy stretch marks
- Sagging fatty buttocks
- Stretch marks of rapid weight increase
- Cellulite
- Sagging inner thighs
- Fatty cushions above knees
- Deformed knees
- Thin skin on legs
- Dry skin on legs
- Muscle atrophy in soles of feet, shoulders, arms, palms of hands,
- Flat feet/reduced arch
- Small breasts in women
- Nervous & anxious behavior
- Tendency to dramatize stressful situations
- Excessive emotional reactions
- Sharp verbal retorts
- Small malar(zygomatic cheek) bones
- Deep nasolabial folds

- Receding gums
- Sagging cheeks
- Jawbone atrophy
- Small chin
- Loose skin folds under chin
- Thin muscles
- Decreased muscle strength
- High systolic and diastolic blood pressure
- Prolonged pinched skin fold
- Muscle atrophy
- Deformed finger joints
- Longitudinal lines on nails
- Poorly developed beard
- Poorly developed chest hair
- Diffuse loss of chest hair
- Small penis/penis atrophy
- Peyronie's disease
- Loose preputium
- Small testicles
- Feels unwell
- Lack of inner peace
- Chronic anxiety without cause

Thymosin Alpha - 1

- Enhances the function of T and dendritic cells immune cells
- Help eradicate the unhealthy cells and stop the infection or cancer growth

Signs of Deficiency

- Looking sick & tired
- Moles all over chest & abdomen
- Warts on hands & feet
- Allergic skin rashes
- Persistent & infected wounds
- Keloids
- Fever blisters on lips
- Erythema of the nose and/or throat
- Fever blisters on genitals
- Mouth ulcers
- Oral or genital herpes
- Lacking drive
- Quickly tired
- Constant bouts of flu
- Recurring herpes
- Acne resistant to other therapies
- Chronic epstein barr virus
- Chronic lyme disease hepatitis b & c
- Hiv infection
- Joint pain
- Constant bouts of disease(joint, intestinal)

Melanotan 2

Signs of Deficiency

- Looks pale (White/caucasian skin)
- Overweight
- Irritable

- Grey, white, red, or blond hair
- Nervous/Anxious behavior
- Flat non curling hair
- Blue Iris
- Pale face
- High blood pressure
- Vitiligo spots
- Women: Clitoral atrophy
- Men: Penile Atrophy
- History of inflammatory diseases in childhood: conjunctivitis, eczema, allergies, celiac disease, etc
- Sexuality that has progressively declined in it's intensity and potency
- Recurring infections as a child
- Learning disabilities
- Low(er) sexual arousal & drive
- Low(er) frequency & Intensity of erotic fantasies
- Low(er) skin sensitivity to sexual caress
- Less sexual arousal
- Less vaginal lubrication
- Difficulties in vaginal opening for penis insertion
- Lower orgasmic capacity
- Erectile Dysfunction: lower frequency and especially duration and strength of erections, less ejaculate volume
- Lower capacities for sexual intercourse
- Permanent silent doubts about sexual capacities and performance
- Possible proneness to infections and inflammation
- Prone to weight gain due to excessive appetite
- Lack of freshness, lack of fresh feeling of being in the spring or on a sunny holiday

- Feeling overworked
- Excess appetite for food
- Flat hair(lack of volume)
- Absent or decrease in curling hair
- Paler hair
- Early greying or whitening of hair
- Blond or red hair
- Difficulty or inability to tan in the sun
- Easily sunburned
- Brittle nails(lacking strength)
- Gastro-enteritis, colitis, celiac disease
- Possible muscle loosening(Multiple sclerosis (MS) may cause a deficiency of GH growth hormone production, particularly in females, who will benefit from either Melanotan 2 or Sermorelin or Tesmorelin to restore muscle firmness and strength.
- Possible joint pain(especially when stressed)
- Note, even one injection could cause a person to look extremely darker than they prefer. Start with a very small dose less than .01 then survey results

Trimix and Quadmix

- Useful in more complicated cases of erectile dysfunction.
- Can potentially restore normal function after one month of use.
- Injections into the penis are helpful in many men where viagra has failed to work; and particularly useful if those men also have clogged arteries.
- The favorite of most porn stars because when used about 30 minutes before making love, the erection can predictably last over one hour or longer..

- It can even help certain paralysis patients who can't make love; however, you need to be very careful with this, and closely guided by your physician, as you can bend or break the penis if you use it incorrectly.
- This combination is becoming less desirable because of the feelings of uncomfortable driving at last sometimes for hours and is distracting do you love making.

Follistatin

- Technically not a peptide but a protein.
- Boosts muscle mass and strength.[10]
- Helps prevent muscle breakdown by inhibiting a protein called myostatin.
- May prevent muscle wasting from aging and neuromuscular disorders.[11]

The Body's Growth Hormone System

Besides Growth hormone (GH) itself, your body utilizes three basic hormones:

---

10 https://www.ncbi.nlm.nih.gov/pmc/articles/PMC2717722/

11 https://www.pnas.org/content/105/11/4318

Are peptides safe? Andrew Huberman https://youtu.be/zU5EYw06wtw?si=5bZ8H7yynvR4KFNi

PEPTIDE MASTERCLASS: The Latest Science Of The Best Peptides For Fat Loss, Muscle & Recovery

https://youtu.be/yKdn6ksVBlk?si=TXA8Xt7UqEev-e86

- **Growth Hormone Releasing Hormone** (GHRH)- Released by the brain to tell your body's growth hormone storage cells (somatotrophs) to release growth hormone.
- **Somatostatin**- Acts as the "off switch" and tells your cells (somatotrophs) to cease growth hormone release.
- **Ghrelin**- Created in the stomach, this hunger derived hormone reduces Somatostatin's "off switch" effect and encourages the brain to release more GHRH.

If GHRH is always around the somatotrophs (GH storing cells) are constantly releasing and unable to store GH. This results in a constant dribble or "bleed" of GH rather than a big pulse. Growing, development, and maturity requires GH to be released in a pulsatile manner.

This is where Somatostatin comes into play. It instructs your somatotrophs to cease the GH release allowing them to begin storing and stockpiling GH. However if Somatostatin is always present the body would never release enough GH to function. What if GHRH and Somatostatin are trying to work at the same time? For the most part Somatostatin is stronger and no GH will be released.

Further benefiting this hormonal seesaw is Ghrelin. When Ghrelin makes its way up to the brain it makes it easier for GHRH to do its job by suppressing Somatostatin's effects. It is possible for Ghrelin on its own to cause a GH release even with a high Somatostatin presence. However, GHRH and Ghrelin together have a synergistic GH effect, meaning that the spike of GH released is larger than could have been produced by each on their own.

Synthetic forms of Ghrelin exist known as Growth Hormone Releasing Peptides (GHRP's) and act in the same way that natural Ghrelin does.

GHRH's

Growth Hormone Releasing Hormones (GHRH):

- CJC-1295*
- CJC-1293
- GRF(1-29)
- Sermorelin
- Modified GRF(1-29)

CJC-1295 is not the same as Mod GRF(1-29)

Which GHRH?

GRF(1-29) and **Sermorelin** are essentially the same thing. Sermorelin is the name of a FDA-approved version of GRF(1-29). The issue here is that these are easily rendered ineffective within minutes of injecting due to destruction by blood enzymes (unless you could pin directly into your pituitary gland). What remains of the list are analogs, or altered versions, of the original GRF(1-29).

Using an analog that is able to survive blood enzymes for around 30 minutes is ideal.

CJC-1293 is GRF(1-29) with 1 amino acid swap plus the Drug Affinity Complex (DAC). DAC acts as a velcro holding the amino acids together for a longer period of time. The single amino acid swap makes the analog peptide stronger but not by enough. The half-life is maybe double GRF(1-29) in humans. So 5 minutes of half-life.

CJC-1295 is GRF(1-29) with 4 amino acid alterations and the Drug Affinity Complex (DAC). This version is extra strong and will last more than 30 minutes and the DAC increases the half-life even more by preventing breakdown by blood enzymes.

Here is the interesting part: you do not want to use any of the CJC's. The first (CJC-1293) does not survive long enough after injection and the second (CJC-1295) survives for too long and is always around preventing Somatostatin from stopping GH release resulting in a GH bleed.

What do you want to use? You want an analog that utilizes those 4 amino acid swaps and maintains the ability to still be broken down after those 30 or so minutes. This is known as **Modified GRF(1-29)**.

GHRP's

Growth Hormone Releasing Peptides, Ghrelin-mimetics (GHRP):

- GHRP-6
- GHRP-2
- Ipamorelin
- Hexarelin

Which GHRP?

GHRP-6 can cause an intense hunger effect and gastric motility. This is a first generation GHRP.

GHRP-2 has a more intense GH release, lower hunger effect, and no gastric motility. GHRP-2 will result in the most bang for your buck. This is a second generation GHRP.

Ipamorelin does not release as much GH as GHRP-2. Has almost no hunger effect.

Schedules under research

Injecting a GHRH on its own is not very effective since you are unable to know when your body's somatostatin is active. Because of this you'll need to pick a GHRP to be paired with your GHRH of choice. This ensures that Somatostatin, if present, will be suppressed and the two peptides will synergistically amplify the natural GH pulse.

Dosing is going to be mostly dependent on your goals and it is generally recommended to assess your tolerance before diving right into multiple doses per day. Starting slow and gradually increasing to multiple doses per day may alleviate some side effects

Note: a saturation dose is defined as 1mcg/kg of bodyweight or 100mcg, the latter being the most commonly used. Some minority of people have sleep interruption rather than better sleep from pre-bed dosing. Often a move from GHRP-6 or GHRP-2 to the smoother Ipamorelin will remedy this. If not, moving the pre-bed dose to the morning often does.

- **Minimalist**- Dosing below saturation levels pre-bed ie: ~50mcg each of a GHRP and GHRH
- **Pre-bed Saturation**- 100mcg of each GHRP and GHRH. Results in better overall health, recovery and well being. This is a solid general anti- aging protocol.
- **Pre-bed & Post Workout Saturation Dose**- PWO using the peptide orally or by injection immediately after the workout serves protein metabolism well and increases protein synthesis. Twice a day saturation doses have increased recovery, contribution to anabolism, injury healing, better well being and serious anti-aging properties.
- **Pre-bed, PWO, and Morning Saturation Doses**- The morning dose, when fasted, engages the release of fatty acids which can be burned off for energy during activity. Three saturation doses per day further increases anabolism and decreases catabolism. Local growth factors will rise including systemic IGF-1, but within physiological levels, resulting in no enhanced health dangers, no abnormal organ or structural growth.

There are more advanced dosing protocols but for simplicity they have been left out of this text.

Administration

For best results, doses should be administered on an empty stomach (approximately 2 hours after eating) or with only plant-based protein. Fats and simple carbs (sugar) blunt the body's GH release.

After administering the dose, wait 20 minutes for the GH pulse to reach its peak. At that point, complex starch-resistant carbohydrates or complex fats (nuts, seeds) can be consumed without worrying about blunting the pulse. If dosing multiple times per day, allow at least 3 hours between meals and peptide administrations.

Safety and Precautions

Peptides are available in supplement form, and when taken orally they are extremely safe. There aren't very many limitations or risks associated with peptide nutraceuticals, so long as you purchase them from a reputable company and take them as directed. See what we believe is the best natural stimulator of peptides:
https://delgadoprotocol.com/product/slimplant-pro/

Peptide injections are also generally considered safe when taken responsibly, which means under the supervision of a good doctor and within the dosage range that is recommended by the manufacturer and your physician. Communication with your healthcare provider is imperative so that they can customize your peptide mixes for maximum benefit.

Contact us at **Delgadolabs.com** or call us at 949-720-1554 and ask for a 15 minute coaching session with one of our experts who can also arrange the doctor to discuss details or prescriptions.

Also, our doctors recommend you start at the minimum suggested dosage, monitor results and effects and adjust accordingly. And finally, if you plan to use injectables make sure the peptides are free of microbes, heavy metals, and other byproducts and actually contain the ingredients advertised. Look for high-quality peptides from a reliable source that has an HPLC lab report; this may cost a bit more but your health is worth it.

Shelf-life and Mixing

As far as shelf-life goes, as long as peptides are stored in a stable condition that is cool and dark and the peptides are not premixed together, most can be stored for years. You can also mix peptides together in one large bottle and draw from that mix. This will allow you to get a cocktail of peptides with just one injection. However, once mixed, the shelf-life is reduced and peptide mixes should be used within a week.

Considerations

When it comes to health, longevity, disease prevention and sexual optimization, you don't want to depend on just one novel therapy. Peptides should be used as an adjunct to a healthy lifestyle. It's important that you also nutrify with a whole foods based diet and nutraceuticals (when necessary); and detoxify with exercise that makes you sweat, proper hydration, a high fiber diet, and liver support. And finally, fortify - by optimizing hormone levels, gut health, stem cell release, mitochondrial function and telomere length.

If you are ready to take control of your health and reverse many of the signs and symptoms of aging, take the Fat Loss and Fitness course. This course guides you through the three proven steps to age reversal - nutrification, detoxification and fortification. It compiles all of the knowledge I have accumulated in over 4 decades of clinical research and practice as a Peak Performance and use Delgado Protocol approved physician It also contains Zee Rak Khan, Love therapist and all of the knowledge and teachings of Susan Bratton, a renowned sex coach. If your main concern is intimacy and lovemaking, we have also collaborated to create an exceptional program. https://foreveryoungevent.com/product/mastering-love-sex-and-intimacy/

These life altering courses on how to enhance Human Performance are priced at this biggest discount, because we love you for a limited time we are offering them both at a massive discount of just $29 each!

And to order the book on Amazon:

https://www.amazon.com/Mastering-Love-Intimacy-Delgado-Ph-D/dp/0996219617

This special offer will not last long, so click on the link above today. foreveryoungevent.com see the section on courses.

Peptides Optimize sexual Energy & body weight.

https://foreveryoungevent.com/product/peptide-procedure/

Our VIP's in monthly coaching received a code for full access. Take this evaluation for a free group session. delgadoprotocol.com/evaluation

Next Apply for Coaching to find out which plan is best for you: https://fromthedoctors.com/services/#perscoach

The tools are emerging. The knowledge is expanding. The future is calling.

It is up to us to use these gifts wisely — to craft a future where vitality is not a privilege of the few, but a birthright of all.

Welcome to the Age of Peptides. Welcome to the future of human potential.

Delgadolabs.com

Sincerely, Nick Delgado, American Board of anti aging health practitioners ABAAHP

"Be Strong Be Well"

About the Author with Academic affiliates

I have strong affiliations with professional and academic organizations, including the American Academy of Anti-Aging Medicine, where I have contributed to blogs for their 35,000 members through publishing articles on their website, leading an online forum for members on A4m.com and Worldhealth.net, and hosting webinars on peptides and estrogen dominance to their members.

I trust this book finds you well in my effort to make you and your loved ones aware of these serious health challenges!

Events Online Summits:

I have participated as a featured presenter at online summits for consumer audiences, including:

foreveryoungevent.com for weekly webinars

As part of our promotional plan for Estrogen Dominance, we ask you to join me as I host more online summits and web classes.

Speaking

I have given over 2,000 talks to live and online audiences with the best of them uploaded to *youtube* and *spotify* search for Beyond Human Dr.NickDelgado on all social media platforms.

It is a lifelong love that helps me pursue my passion for helping people improve their health, one that will only intensify in my support of this book and my audience.

I am a regular speaker at the five largest health expos, which are also streamed online, increasing their reach exponentially:

- Whole Life Expo
- New Life Expo in San Francisco

- LA Conscious Life Expo
- TheRealTruthaboutHealth.com
- New Paradigm Shift Conference
- SoCal VegFest
- WorldHealth.net
- A4m.com
- bio hacking events

See my coming events at entrepreneur groups and every Monday afternoon and Wednesday night at Dr. Nick Delgado schedule at *foreveryoungevent.com* via *restream, youtube, facebook*

Tuesday I cover the subjects related to **Acne be Gone for Good**

I also regularly present at or attend academic conferences, including:

- The British Society of-Anti-Aging Medicine's Annual Anti-Aging Conference
- Anti Aging Academy Anti Aging Congress
- American Academy of-Anti-Aging Medicine

Publishing Track Record

Author of multiple books, including:

Stop Aging Now *- 7 Secrets to Look & Feel Great Forever* by Nick Delgado, Board Certified ABAAHP (2023)

Blood Doesn't Lie by Dr. Nick Delgado, ABAAHP (2020)

Mastering Love Sex and Intimacy by Dr. Nick Delgado copyright (2019)

Acne be Gone for Good (2018)-by-SoniaBadreshia Bansal,MD,FAAD,Board Certified Dermatologist, Nick Delgado, ABAAHP, ***Annihilate Acne Naturally*** (2016), recipient of the **Irwin award for best health book** by Book Publicists of Southern California, a guide to making the dietary and lifestyle changes that no traditional dermatologist will tell you to cure this emotionally and physically scarring epidemic. This self-published book has reached a growing audience of loyal fans.

Simply Healthy (2012), a cookbook that features plant-based recipes that follow the Delgado Protocol. When attendees review through this picture filled example of tasty recipes they invest in getting a copy of this easy to follow recipe book.

Stem Cells for Joint Fitness Plus anti-aging methods to feel great, be fit and pain-free by anti-aging expert and fitness star Nick Delgado PhD (2010) written for health professionals.

Grow Young and Slim. Overcome obesity and poor health with a startling Concept that will break through all the myths on Aging by Nick Delgado PhD and Shawn Kendell (2000) This is still a very popular book because it covers hormones, diet, exercise, as a cornerstone to health.

How to Look great and feel Sexy- Revitalize your energy in 9 days over 600 recipes Nick Delgado m.s, Ph.D (1997)

Mastering the Powers of Your Inner Health. How to utilize natural abilities to consistently produce Peak Performance levels of Maximum energy and health also the latest on nutrition for pregnancy infants and children by Nicholas Delgado (1992)

Weight Loss and Energy Now *(1992)*
fatigue to vitality (1991) by Nick Delgado PhD

Online Product Sales

- **EstroBlock.com**
  This website is where I house all content and products that relate to the subject of estrogen dominance. I will create a presence here for *Estrogen Dominance* as part of the book launch campaign.

DelgadoProtocol.com/Hub

A site that offers our best supplements that also include natural herbal combinations specific to solving estrogen dominance, with over 200 health professionals and over 2,000 individuals and buyers who purchase supplements from our websites and amazon.com. We offer gifts and donations to worthy causes for kids and families struggling with autism, cancer and chronic diseases of aging.

We expect to grow exponentially as our best selling product EstroBlock ships to more countries. Currently, three of our products have been accepted by Canada. We are now focusing on our newest release **EstroBlock** both Pro and **Vitality** into Asia, Indonesia, Australia, Germany and the U.K.

Several vendors have asked us to share our books and product list informing new customers of *Estroblock.com* as part of this newest book campaign.

to locate the best Peptides go to delgadolab.com

- **foreveryoungevent.com**
- My main mentoring and the coaching website foreveryoungevent.com where we have created a series of online courses*
- visit Amazon for **audible** kindle books search books by Dr. Nick Delgado

Social Media Presence

- Youtube.com/delgadovideo
- YouTube channel, youtube.com/delgadoprotocol where I release one to two videos per week (We have 2,200 already completed and organized into playlists that cover most health challenges you and your family may encounter during life's journey.
- We are excited to announce short form videos on our EstroBlock channel:
- https://youtube.com/@estroblockshorts?si=5kdpOjO0WEzGxWYm
- We can be found on most social media platforms located as Dr. Nick Delgado
- Instagram
  @estroblockprotocol: 27,000 followers

- X-Twitter
  @delgadoprotocol: 1600 followers

Media

I'm excited to appear on many popular outlets, as I've been a guest on several shows:

- Ben Greenfield Fitness, podcast host and author of bestselling book *Beyond Training,* whose website gets over 250,000 monthly visitors.
- The Dr. Drew podcast
- David Snow podcast
- Chef AJ
- Frankie Boyer, radio talk show host
- James Lowe, radio talk show host
- Late Night Health podcast with Marc Alyn

Marketing and Publicity

I believe the release of this book is spreading effectively by word of mouth and influencers who invite me onto their podcasts and talk shows.

Please contact us at Nick@delgadoprotocol.com and DM me on instagram Dr.NickDelgado

Call us at 949-720-1554. M-F 10 am to 4 pm PST. Text us at 949-913-0000 or whatsapp

We love you and thank you for your thoughtful engagement on social media, amazon and google comments.

Book Titles that motivated me to write this book

Defeat Estrogen Toxins will appeal to readers of other successful works that help them restore balance to their hormones to regulate their weight, relieve chronic conditions, and promote their overall vitality.

With a hormone-balance protocol developed by an impeccably credentialed physician—as well as complementary supplements and other products—the closest comparisons are *The Hormone Reset Diet: Heal Your Metabolism to Lose Up to 15 Pounds in 21 Days* by Sara Gottfried, M.D., a *New York Times* bestseller released in March 2016, and *The Hormone Cure,* Gottfried's previous book released in 2013. A distinction between *my book* and *The Hormone Reset Diet* is that my book focuses on estrogen and its related hormonal imbalance, making the message simpler and easier to integrate into the readers' lives. Unlike *The Hormone Cure, Estrogen Dominance* speaks to both men and women. It's a book that the whole family can benefit from.

Mark Hyman's books, *The Blood Sugar Solution 10-Day Detox Diet*—which debuted in the number one spot on both the Amazon and *New York Times* bestseller lists—and *The Blood Sugar Solution*—which was a seven-time *New York Times* bestseller—combine research, supplements, and diet modifications that provide far-reaching health benefits.

The Plant Paradox Dr Steven Gundry MD 16,327 reviews

Estrogeneration-How Estogenics are Making you Fat, Sick and Infertile by Anthony G Jay PhD reviews

Overcoming Estrogen Dominance by Magdalena Wszelaki 343 reviews

The Anti-Estrogenic Diet by Ori Hofmekler 252 reviews

The Great Cholesterol Myth, Revised and Expanded Why lowering.. By Jonny Bowden 1,567 reviews

... Ken Berry 7,111 reviews

Gut and Psychology Syndrome: Natural Treatments for Autism by Natasha Campbell-McBride 2,664 reviews As a parent of a child diagnosed with learning difficulties, she was acutely aware of the difficulties facing other parents like her, and she has devoted much of her time to helping these families. She realized that nutrition played a critical role in helping children and adults to overcome their disabilities, and has pioneered the use of probiotics in this field.

***The Way of the Superior Man by David Deida 13,936 reviews Summary & Review*

Find Your Life's Purpose.

Embrace Your Masculine Energy: Polarization Attracts.

Embrace Her Drama.

For Real Passion: Let Go, Ravish Her.

Leverage Sexual Energy: Don't Come.

Face Your Fears, Do Your Best (& Get Friends Who Do The Same)

The Life Plan How Any Man Can Achieve Lasting Health, Great Sex and by Jeffry Life MD PhD 507 reviews

Optimize your health peptides Extend your life by being more muscular, leaner, smarter, injury free and younger Jay Campbell 387 reviews

The Changing World Order Ray Dalio 7,832 reviews

The 4 hour Body: An Uncommon Guide to by Timothy Ferriss 8,946 reviews

Good Energy by Casey Means MD

Boundless upgrade your Brain & Defy Aging Ben Greenfield 2,144 reviews

The Testosterone Optimization Therapy Bible by Jay Campbell 636 reviews

Testosterone for Life A Morgentaler 411 reviews

Estrogen Dominance Hormonal Imbalance of the 21st Century Michael Lam (59 reviews

The End of the World is just the beginning Peter Zehan 4,887 reviews

12 Rules of Life Jordan Pederson 81,000 reviews

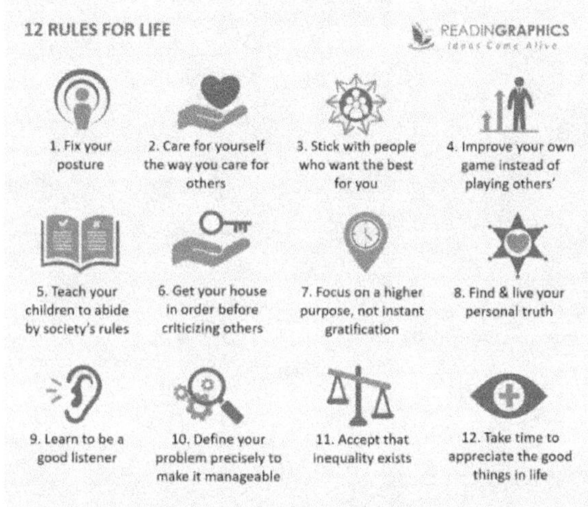

Why we get sick Benjamin Bikman 3,800 reviews

Estrogen Matters Avrum Bluming 726 reviews

Iodine David Brownstein 374 reviews

Why We Sleep Matthew Walker 32,000 reviews

A Poison Like no Other How microplastics corrupted our planet Matt Simon 38 reviews

Defeat Estrogen Toxins

Nick Delgado *shares a singular focus on a particular disease culprit but differentiates itself by talking about a particular* aspect of health that none of the biggest voices in natural health have addressed yet.

www.ingramcontent.com/pod-product-compliance
Lightning Source LLC
LaVergne TN
LVHW010916110826
845149LV00013B/2382

* 9 7 9 8 9 9 3 0 3 7 0 3 5 *